GEORGE COUNTY HOSPITAL

HOSPITAL

the first 50 years

Wyatt House books may be ordered through booksellers or by contacting:

WYATT HOUSE PUBLISHING
399 Lakeview Dr. W.
Mobile, Alabama 36695
www.wyattpublishing.com
editor@wyattpublishing.com

Because of the dynamic nature of the Internet, any web address or links contained in this book may have changed since publication and may no longer be valid.

Cover and interior design by: Mark Wyatt

ISBN 13: 978-1-7326049-8-8

Printed in the United States of America

CONTENTS

The Committee

Dr. Dayton Whites

Joyce Rutherford

Patsy Smith

Christine Davis

Patricia Howell

Tabatha Pinter

Christy Pope

Christy Roberts

Deryk Parker

Belva Hayden

Derrick Scott

Carman Walley Cochran

Stephanie Chisholm

Faye McNeil

Kathryn Cooley

Andria Dees

Introduction

Someone once said, "When a person is buried at the end of life, buried with them is an entire encyclopedia of events." This has been proven true during the writing of this book. We have diligently striven to recover information on the first 50 years of George County Hospital. If it had been possible to retrieve the information lost before former employees passed, this would be a great book.

Early in 2019, a group of present and former employees came together with the idea of putting together a small book covering the first 50 years of George County Hospital. This period covers the beginning of the hospital during a time when the hospital was small and employees felt like members of a close-knit family who ran the hospital. The story we tell here ends in the year 2000 when the hospital became larger and moved into the 21st century.

Each unit of the book was written by a person either presently working in that department or who had worked in that department before. Other information was gathered from the best sources available to us.

Every effort was made to ensure the accuracy of the information in this book. Please excuse any mistakes.

History of George County Hospital

In 1947, George County did not have a hospital facility. The only thing resembling the hospital was a former residence located on Main Street, which was called "the birthing house". Here Dr. McMillan and Dr. Horn admitted women in labor. They had a registered nurse by the name of Pauline Parker follow the patients through labor. One of the physicians would deliver the baby and discharge the mother and baby the following morning.

In 1947 George County patients were seen mostly on house calls or in the physician's office. Patients needing hospitalization were sent to Mobile, Pascagoula or Hattiesburg for treatment.

Over several years leading up to 1947, the George County Board of Supervisors began putting aside money in a fund called "the hospital fund". Beat one supervisor, Grady Younge had headed up this program. In 1947 there was approximately $74,000 set aside for this purpose.

A bill had passed in the Federal Congress in 1946 called the Hill Burton act. The purpose of this bill was to allow the federal government, along with the state government, to help finance the cost of building a hospital the local government could not afford to build. In this bill, the rural hospital cost would be split three ways. Federal money would be one third, state money would be one third and the local government would supply the final one third.

George County's application for Hill Burton fund was approved. The federal government approved $88,104. The State of Mississippi paid $107,705, and George County added its $74,406.

In December 1947 with the money available, George County Board of Supervisors moved forward with the project. Property was purchased on Winter Street from the William Thomas family. Vincent Smith was hired as the architect.

Cost of the new hospital was as follows: land $6902, architect $8385, equipment $41,692, site survey $363, title search, $1000 construction cost $209,640, and supervision during construction $4192.

George County's Hill Burton Hospital would be a modern 35 bed hospital with an operating room, a delivery room, a laboratory, x-ray department, emergency room, administrative office, and a mechanic room. The property would be landscaped and have a paved parking area.

On September 2, 1950 George County Hospital opened its doors to treat patients. The first medical staff consisted of Dr. A.K. McMillan, Dr. John Horn, Dr. J. K. Spiceland, Dr. Raymond Benson, Dr. Lit Eubanks, Dr. S. H. McDonniel and Dr. Millard Jensen.

Mr. John Lumpkin was chairman of the first George County Hospital board. A registered nurse by the name of Mae Whitlow was named hospital superintendent.

Patient's cost for use of the hospital was very low. Hospital room rates were $10 per day, laboratory procedures were $2-3 dollars, x-rays were $10-$12 and OB care for a delivery was approximately $90-$100. This included a three-day hospital stay after delivery. Major surgery charges were very similar to OB charges.

The hospital was well accepted by the people in the George County area. In July 1952 George County Hospital became a member of the Mississippi State Hospital Association. That same year, Blue Cross Blue Shield began paying for hospital usage by their customers. In 1954, George County Hospital was air-conditioned.

In 1959, because of use of the patients of this area, more beds were needed. On the south end of the hospital, plans were made to add an additional nine private rooms. Also there would be a nurse's station placed in this area. This addition would cost approximately $20,000 and be called the McMillan addition in honor of Dr. A. K. McMillan. This addition was opened in 1960.

A second addition would be added in 1964. This was during Mr. Keith Scott's time as hospital administrator. The cost of this addition would be approximately $80,000 and would include a new entrance, waiting area, newborn nursery, 4 OB beds and 7 semiprivate rooms. This addition opened in 1960 and would be called the Keith Scott addition.

In 1964, George County Hospital installed telephones in all hospital rooms.

In the mid 1970's, there was a major construction project at George County Hospital. This included the addition of E. R waiting room and office, C. C. U. and Intensive care unit and enlargement of the Laboratory and X ray Department. Surgery would be moved and recovery room added. Two labor rooms would be added. Sterile and unsterile areas would be improved. Numerous other improvements were made.

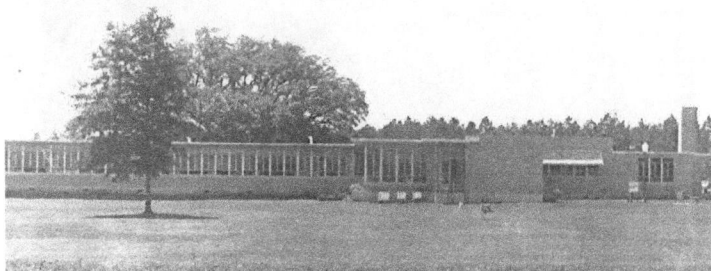

George County Hospital, 1950

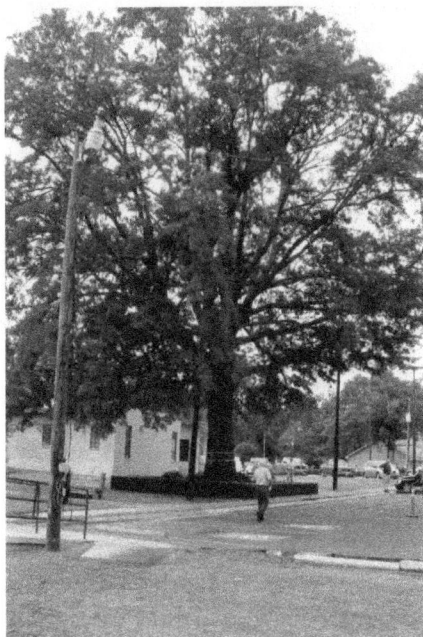

Recognize the tree?

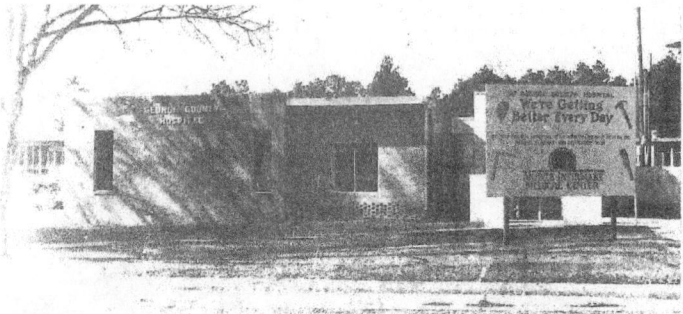

Name Change... THE GEORGE COUNTY Hospital in Lucedale is changing its name to the George County Infirmary. This name change was suggested by the hospital's Advisory Board and approved by the State Department of Health, Division of Licenses and Certifications this past week.

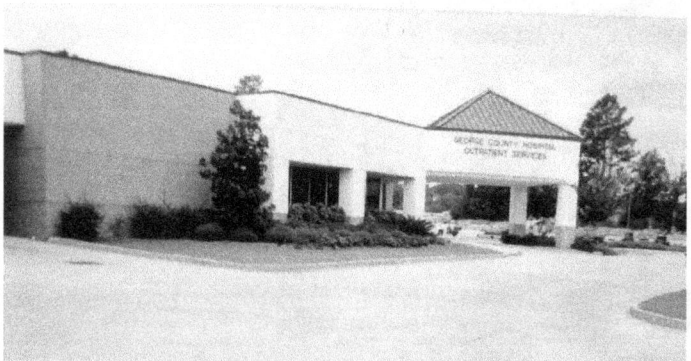

George County Hospital Outpatient

In 1985, after several short-term administrators, George County Board of Supervisors decided they would lease the hospital to an outside group. Against the advice of the medical staff, the hospital was leased to Gulf Health Systems. During their four years of management of George County Hospital, they constructed an elaborate, covered walkway at the main entrance, a small doctors' lounge, and additional space in the administration area. This lease did not work well and was canceled after 4 years.

Once management of George County Hospital was returned to the George County Board of Supervisors, the Board appointed a new hospital Board of Trustees. They quickly appointed Mrs. Kathryn Cooley as interim hospital administrator. She served for a year and did well. She asked to be replaced.

Several qualified administrators would serve over the next four years. In 1993, Mr. Paul Gardner was hired as hospital administrator. With a shared vision, Mr. Gardner and the board began to make plans for a hospital addition.

This addition would be started by the year 2000, but not completed until later. The new addition would be designed to handle increased demand for outpatient care. The new building would also increase the size of the surgery department and add new patient rooms, a new intensive care unit, an OB suite, emergency rooms, and most of all, an outpatient area with a large waiting room.

Board of Trustees

The first Board of Trustees for George County Hospital consisted of John Lumpkin, president, Charles Holland, R. H. Persons, Donald Vincent, and Coleman Rouse.

The book containing the minutes of the George County Hospital board meetings has been destroyed. It has been suggested, that in the early 80' the book was damaged by water and disposed of. This book would have contained the names of the board members.

Through research, where information was available, these are the names of persons, who have served on the George County Hospital board. They will be divided into three groups. The first group, will be those who served from the opening of the hospital until 1985. From 1985 to 1989, Mobile Infirmary ran the hospital. Dr. Victor Landry was one of the members of the local advisory board, no other names were available. The last group is composed of those members who served from 1989 to the year 2000.

The names of the first group include those listed on the first George County Hospital board listed above and the following - J. F. Averett, Charles Howell, Roy Grafe, Ray Havard, Everett O'Neal, Jimmy Vise, James Whittington, Linton Moore, and Byford Mallette. The last group would include Cecilia Cochran, Brenda Collins, Margaret Dixon, Burton Flurry, Lester Hatcher, Simmie Hollinghead, Jeff Howell, Stephen Maples, Gary Spooner and Mendell Wachsman.

We realize it is very likely someone's name has been left out. We apologize, but this is the best list our research has given us.

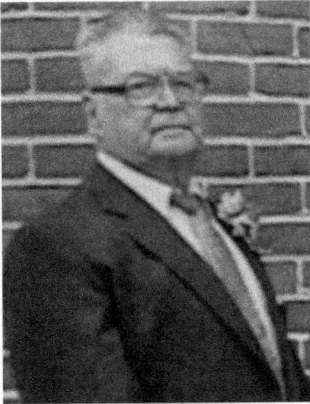

Coleman Rouse

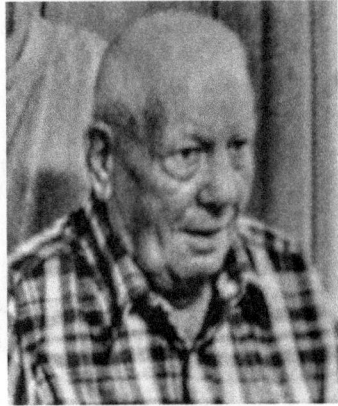

Don Vincent

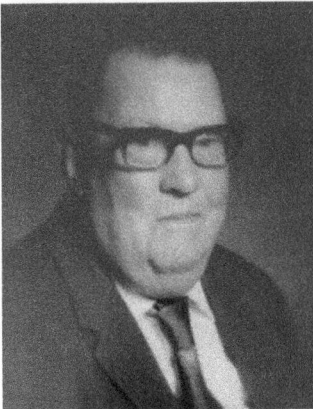

Charles Holland

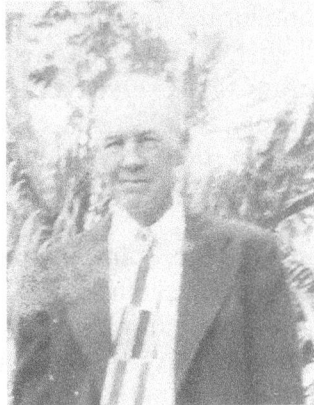

John Lumpkin
First Chairman of the Board

Administrators

George County Hospital opened in September, 1950. The hospital board hired Mrs. Mae Whitlow from Op, Alabama as superintendent of the hospital. She was a registered nurse. She served in that position, until 1954. At that time, Dr. A.K. McMillan was Chief of the Medical Staff and he assumed the responsibility as hospital administrator for the next two years.

In 1956 a local registered nurse, Mrs. Hazel Croom became the Hospital Administrator. She served in this position for the next six years. Mr. Keith Scott, hospital anesthetist, was hired as Hospital Administrator to replace her in 1961. He served as administrator until his resignation in 1964. Mr. Douglas Mixon served for a short period of time in 1964. That same year, Mr. Scott was rehired for an additional four years.

In 1968 Mr. Johnny Mills was hired as hospital administrator. He served in that position until his resignation in 1976. Mr. Lowell Benton would serve as the next administrator. In 1981, Mr. B. L. Lott would serve for one year. Mr. Lewis Smith followed Mr. Lott. He would serve from 1981 through 1984.

In 1984, because of the dissatisfaction of the George County Board of Supervisors with the hospital, it would be leased to Mobile Infirmary Hospital in Mobile, Alabama. This lease was not satisfactory. However, it lasted for approximately four years. During this period of time, there were two hospital administrators. One was Mr. Rupert Ingram, who served from 1985 to 1988 and Mr. Jim Hudnall, who served 1988 and 1989.

George County Board of Supervisors took the hospital back over in 1989. They appointed Kathryn Cooley as interim Administrator for a period of one year. Mr. Robert Hughes was hired as Hospital Administrator in 1990 and was replaced by Paul Harris, interim administrator for several months.

In 1991, Ted Lorentz was appointed administrator by the hospital board. He served for two years and was replaced in 1993, by Mr. Paul Gardner, who would be administrator through the year 2015.

Administration

George County Hospital has had approximately 20 hospital administrators. We have attempted to contact all the past administrators and have asked for information about their years at George County Hospital.

Only three administrators have replied. These are Mr. Johnny Mills (1968-1976), Kathryn Cooley (1989-1991) and Mr. Paul Gardner (1993-2015).

Johnny Mills and Paul Gardner were the longest-serving administrators and much was accomplished during their time at George County Hospital.

George County Hospital:

1968-1976

In April 1968, Johnny Mills was appointed Hospital Administrator by the Hospital's board of five trustees. The trustees' names were Don Vincent, Charles Holland, Everett O'neal, J.F. Averett, and C.C. Rouse. Bill Bailey was the Hospital's attorney. Horace Bradley was the Hospital's independent accountant.

The mission of the Hospital's trustees and medical staff was to maintain the Hospital's highest standards for relieving pain and suffering. The medical staff consisted of Dr. Whites, Dr. Tipton, Dr. Shaw, Dr. Gonzalez, Dr. Landry, and Dr. Eubanks. The Surgery department staff consisted of Keith Scott, anesthetist, Lena Wozencraft, RN, Corine Morgan, LPN. Ms. Mattie Terry, and Ms. Izola Miles worked as sterile supply technicians. It was not unusual for the surgeons, assisting doctors, and operating room staff to work twelve or more hours each day.

During Mills' eight years as administrator, the Hospital's capacity was sixty beds plus the nursery. During the flu and other epidemic seasons, beds were put in the hallways and lobby for treating patients.

The following thoughts are contributed by Johnny Mills:

I believe it was in 1970 that a patient came up missing.

17

The Hospital staff, city police, and the sheriff's department were all looking everywhere for the missing patient. At this time, the George County Rebels were playing football about three blocks from the Hospital. After the game was over, one of the Hospital employees came running up to me with news that the patient was walking the hallway going to his room. His excuse for slipping out of the Hospital was, "I have never missed a football game when the Rebels were playing." What a relief it was to have the patient back in his hospital bed!

In 1971, a bedside-to-nurse-station call system was installed. This gave the patient an immediate contact for needed services.

In 1972, the Board of Trustees approved the first personnel policies. This action was taken for consistency in managing the Hospital's employees.

In 1972, a chapel was added to the Hospital. This would give the patients and their families, along with the hospital staff, a place to worship and find peace with their Lord.

In March of 1973, the Hospital Board of Trustees accepted the community's request to operate an ambulance service. The trustees and medical staff wholeheartedly supported the request.

On September 6, 1973, the Hospital and Glen Oaks Nursing Home sponsored the first certified practical nursing (LPN) school. Eleven students received their LPN certificates. The graduation exercise was at the fairly new George County Occupational Training Center.

In 1974, a major addition to the Hospital got underway. It consisted of an intensive care unit, operating rooms, anesthesia department, recovery room, inhalation therapy department, labor room for expectant mothers, and enlargement of the sterile supply, laboratory, and x-ray departments. A waiting room for outpatients was also added.

George County Hospital

1989-1991

By Kathryn Cooley

Jim Hudnall was the Administrator of George County Hospital in the late 1980's. The Hospital was nearing the end of its contract with Mobile Infirmary.

Board members asked me, the D.O.N., to be interim administrator. The board of trustees was eager to assist and make recommendations for the Hospital. Eventually, I requested the board of trustees find a permanent administrator for the Hospital.

Major Issues From 1991 to 2000

By Paul Gardner, CEO

The Horne CPA firm brought me from Jackson, Ms. to Lucedale in September 1990. Horne CPA performs a lot of Healthcare work and George County Hospital was a client. I was performing accounting work for the hospital, which was having some very serious financial troubles at the time. Most suppliers had placed the hospital on cash on delivery (COD) status.

In the spring of 1991, I met with the George County Board of Supervisors to inform them that if changes were not made, the hospital was facing possible closure. A few months later, the Supervisors approached me about coming to work for the hospital to help fix the financial problems.

Shortly after arriving at George County Hospital, I learned that one of the main physicians in town, Dr. Tom Shaw, had been diagnosed with cancer and had been given only a few months to live. This situation dealt a major blow to the community and especially to an already stressed hospital and medical practice, leaving only his partner, Dr. Dayton Whites to manage patients.

This situation prompted the hospital in George County to purchase their practice, Community Medical Center, which was the major health clinic in town in 1992. This move would help to secure the hospital's future and recruit more physicians to town. The hospital would later acquire the other two medical practices in town, owned by Dr. Victor Landry and Dr. Daniel Gonzalez.

In 1996, George County Hospital, with the help of a Rural Outreach Grant, opened a medical clinic in the Greene County Hospital building, which had recently closed. This was our neighbor to the north and part of our market area. They were in desperate need of healthcare in that county.

In 1998, we reimplemented Obstetrical services at George County Hospital, after being shut down for several years. Delivering babies again at our hospital was gladly received by the community. That same year we purchased the old Greer's strip mall structure. The Hospital system converted most of that space to accommodate visiting specialists and opened the county's first Wellness Center. We moved our Rehab department over to that facility and renamed it "Southeast Rehab Center".

In 1999, we were able to add Ear, Nose and Throat services with the addition of Rufus Neel, MD to our medical staff. He was a Lucedale boy who had traveled all over the world practicing medicine. He was well received by the community. His practice was placed in the old Dr. Gonzalez building, which the hospital had purchased.

With the help of a Bond Issue passed by the County Supervisors, we were able to add 30,000 square feet to the hospital facility. This included a new Emergency Department, a six bed Intensive Care Unit, an Out-Patient Surgery Suite, a new Labor and Delivery Suite and eight new patient rooms with a new nurse's station. We were able then to renovate some of the old space to improve our lab and doctors' lounge.

This project also included a new 21,000 square foot Medical Office building. The old Community Medical Center building was utilized to house visiting specialists from out of town. This project helped to modernize an old Hill-Burton Hospital in serious need of updating and expansion.

Construction was completed in the 2000's. The new surgery space allowed us to add additional services such as orthopedics, ophthalmology and dental. Along with general surgery, we now had ENT and OB/GYN cases. Our surgery volumes greatly increased. Upon completion of the construction project and over the next several years, we were able to attract and recruit several physicians, including Family Practice, Internal Medicine, pediatricians and OB/GYN. The addition of new space and new physicians vastly improved the community's opinion of the local hospital and improved utilization of it.

These developments, along with the implementation of good business strategies, placed the George County Hospital on sound footing.

In 2000, we worked with Dr. Bobby Burn from Wiggins, MS to open a medical clinic in that town. Dr. Burn was well liked and performed endoscopes at our hospital, which also added to our volumes.

By the year 2000, George County Hospital was doing very well financially and in the area of care it delivered.

The system added a nursing home to the George County facility and took over the Greene County Hospital and Greene County Nursing Home and Clinic in the early 2000's. Over this period, we developed into a small regional healthcare system, serving three counties.

Administrators

GREG HAVARD	2015-PRESENT
PAUL GARDNER	1993-2015
TED LORENZ, JR	1991-1993
PAUL HARRIS	1991
ROBERT HUGHES	1990-1991
KATHRYN COOLEY	1989-1990
JAMES HUDNALL	1988-1989
GULF HEALTH SYSTEM	1985-1988
RUPERT INGRAM	1985-1988
LOWELL BENTON	1984-1985
LEWIS SMITH	1981-1984
KEITH SCOTT, Interim	1980-1981
B.L. LOTT	1976-1980
JOHNNY MILLS	1968-1976
KEITH SCOTT	1964-1968
DOUG MIXON	1964
KEITH SCOTT	1961-1964
HAZEL CROOM	1956-1961
DR. McMILLIAN	1954-1956
MAE WHITLOW	1950-1954

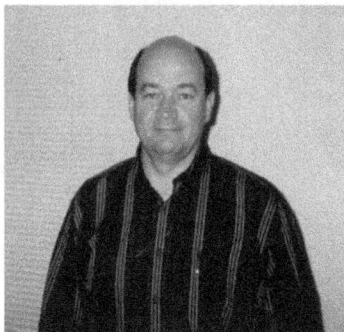

Paul Gardner

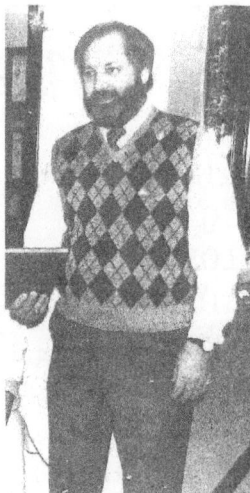

Rupert Ingram

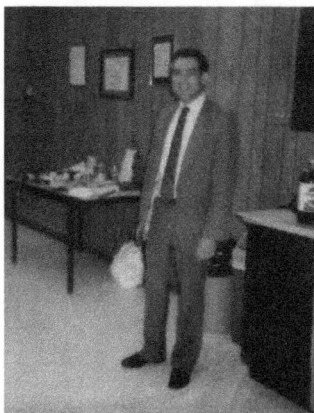

Jim Hudnall

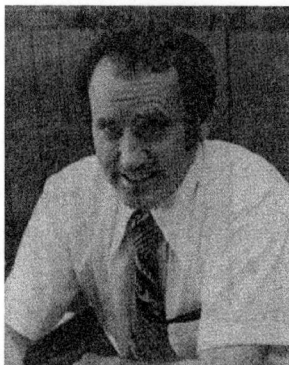

Johnny Mills

Physicians

on the medical staff of George County Hospital

1950- 2000

By Dr. Dayton Whites

On September 2, 1950, George County Hospital opened its doors to serve the people in George County and the surrounding areas. The first medical staff consisted of the following physicians.

1. Dr. A. K. McMillan: Died in 1968.

2. Dr. J. L. Spiceland: Died in 1955.

3. Dr. J. W. Horn: Died in 1956.

4. Dr. Raymond Benson: Killed in an automobile accident in 1955.

5. Dr. S. H. McDonniel: Left Lucedale in 1955 to be student physician at University Medical Center.

6. Dr. L. H. Eubanks: Retired in 1977. He was also a very active farmer in George County.

7. Dr. Millard Jensen: Left Lucedale in 1960. He was a local who had a very active practice and served two years of active duty in the Army National Guard while practicing in Lucedale.

Listed below are the physicians who have served on George County Hospital medical staff:

1. Dr. L.B. Hudson (1951) was a general practitioner. No information is available.

2. Dr. R.B. Izzard (1952-1956) was a general practitioner. Prior to coming to Lucedale, he was a physician on an Indian reservation. He was married to one of the R. M. McKay daughters. He returned to serve as a physician on an Indian reservation after practicing in Lucedale.

3. Dr. Victor Landry (1953-1999) was a general practitioner and surgeon. He moved here from Collins, Mississippi. He was an excellent doctor and probably was on the medical staff longer than any other medical staff member.

4. Dr. Raymond Tipton (1954-1993) was a general practitioner. He was an outstanding diagnostician. He was a local who returned to Lucedale to practice as a general practitioner. He was also very involved in sports at George High School.

5. Dr. Louis Rittamyer (1953-1955). He was a general practitioner and a very delightful person, who smiled all the time, which caused patients to feel that he did not have proper concern for their illness and pain.

6. Dr. Daniel Gonzales (1960-1996) was a general practitioner and general surgeon. He had a very active practice. He was good. He married a local girl, Martha Skinner.

7. Dr. Dayton Whites (1961-1999). He was a hometown boy and board-certified family physician. He loved the practice of medicine and his patients. He also served as mayor of Lucedale 2001- 2009.

8. Dr. Thomas Shaw (1964-1991) was an excellent board-certified family physician. He had good medical judgment and gave his patients excellent care. He died prematurely in 1991 from lung cancer.

9. Dr. George Orndorff (1978-1980) was a general practitioner who came to Lucedale under a federal program for underserved medical areas.

10. Dr. Skip Brister (1983-1985) was a general practitioner who did well in his practice. He went to Hurley for a short time and later went into psychiatry.

11. Dr. Herbert Kinsey (1975-1980) was a board-certified general surgeon. He was also a part of Community Medical Center and an excellent surgeon. Prior to coming to Lucedale, he practiced in Central Alabama and returned to his previous location upon leaving Lucedale. He was married to local girl, Mary Stonecypher.

12. Dr. John Bearry (1979-1980) was a general practitioner and a local who returned to Lucedale to practice

medicine. He was super smart and had an outstanding ability to care for critically ill patients.

13. Dr. John Campbell (1986-1988) was a general practitioner and moved to Lucedale partially because he had married a Lucedale girl. He was very independent in his practice of medicine.

14. Dr. Suresh Chintamaneni (1988-1997) was a general surgeon. He was originally from India. Undoubtedly, he was the most qualified and best surgeon George County had ever had. He made a great contribution to medicine and surgery during his nine years at George County Hospital.

15. Dr. William Bennett (1991-1993) was a board certified internist with special training in gastroenterology. He was a good doctor and contributed a great deal during the loss of Dr. Shaw. He died prematurely of myocardial infarction while practicing on an Indian reservation.

16. Dr. Richard Cunningham (1990-1996) was a general practitioner and moved here from Wiggins Mississippi. He loved his patients and got very involved with their care. He was also very important during the loss of Dr. Shaw.

17. Dr. Tara Mallette (1992-2016) was a local girl who returned to Lucedale as a board-certified pediatrician.

She gave excellent care to pediatric patients. She is a member of the Scott family, most of whom are medical professionals.

18. Dr. Rufus Neel (1992-2009) was a board certified ENT plastic surgeon. He was a local boy who returned to his hometown. He was more than excellent in his field of ENT.

19. Dr. Harilal Patel (1993-2016) was certified in Internal Medicine. He was an excellent physician and added much to medicine in George County.

20. Dr. Seth Scott (1994-present) was a board-certified family physician and was very important in the practice and management of Community Medical Center. He and Dr. Tara Mallette are siblings.

21. Dr. Kevin O'Hea (1996-2011) was a family physician. He came to Lucedale from Canada. He was an excellent physician and contributed very much to Community Medical Center and to medicine in George County.

22. Dr. Michael Huber (1997-present) was a board certified family physician. He was another great Dr. who is an excellent diagnostician and gave excellent care to his patients. He remains important to Community Medical Center and the patients of George County.

23. Dr. Kornstein (1996-1999) was an OBGYN specialist. He reestablished delivering of babies at George County Hospital (GCH).

24. Denise Teasley (1998-2008) OB/GYN specialist. Excellent physician, she raised the standard of women's care at George County Hospital.

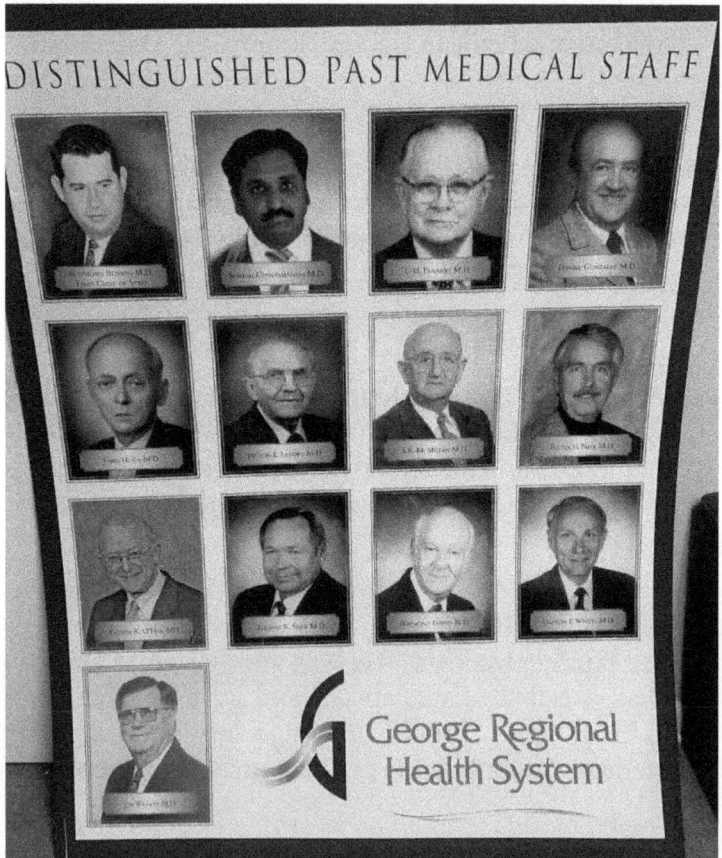

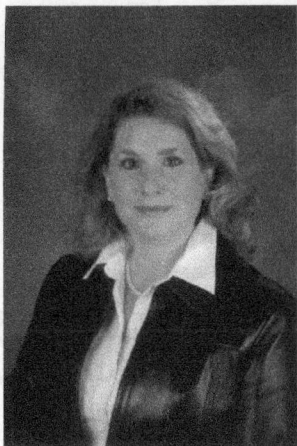

Dr. Tara Mallett

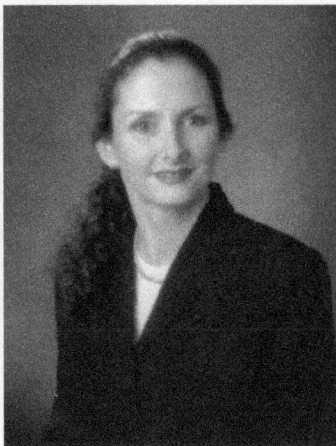

Dr. Denise Teasley

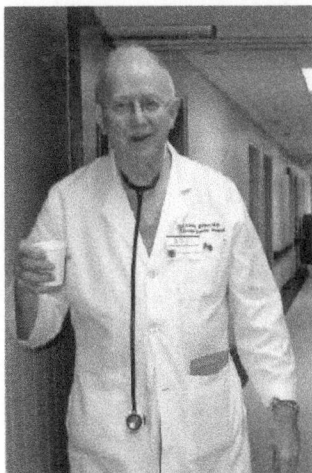

Dr. Kevin O'Hea

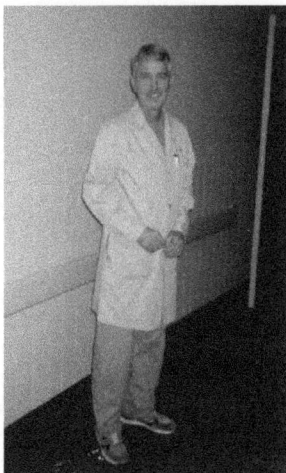

Dr. Neel

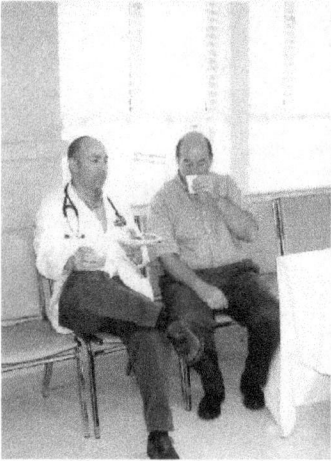

Dr. Huber and Paul Gardner

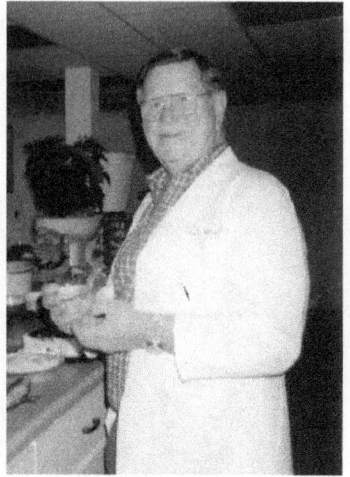

Dr. Wilhite

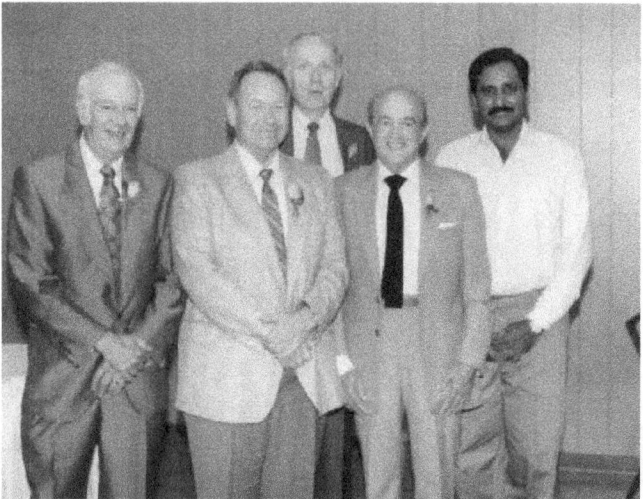

l-r: Dr. Tipton, Dr. Shaw, Dr. Whites,
Dr. Gonzalez, Dr. Suresh

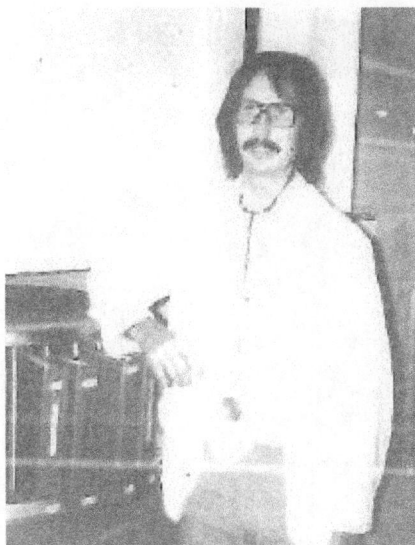

Dr. John Bearry

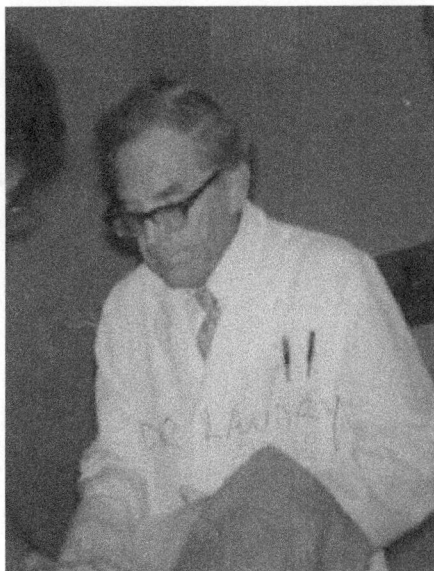

Dr. Landry

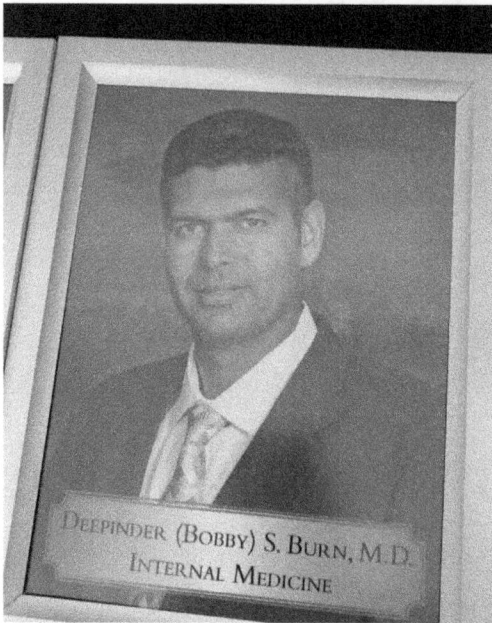

Deepinder (Bobby) S. Burn, M.D.
Internal Medicine

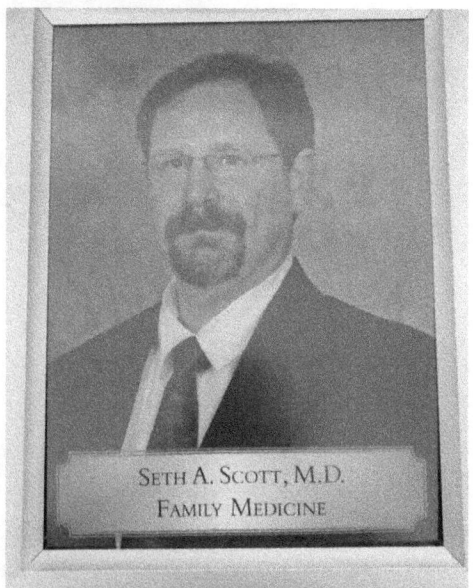

Seth A. Scott, M.D.
Family Medicine

Surgery Department: First 50 Years

By Belva Hayden and Derrick Scott

George County Hospital has a long and proud history of providing surgical care to the people of George County. Surgical services have been provided from the beginning. Dr. Raymond Benson, Dr. Victor Landry, and Dr. Lit H. Eubanks provided most of the surgical care in the early years. This was the era of the general practitioners who were trained to do everything from treating diabetes to delivering babies.

With the advancements in healthcare, particularly in surgical specialty, many well-trained surgeons started arriving in the 1960s. Dr. Daniel Gonzalez arrived in 1960 and practiced general surgery at GCH until 1996.

Dr. Herbert Kinsey and Dr. Dewey Lane were on staff at GCH in the 1970s and 80s. Dr. Suresh Chintamaneni arrived in 1989 and provided excellent surgical and emergency care for the people of George County until 1997.

Dr. Rufus Neel was born and raised in Lucedale and moved back home in 1995 to practice ear, nose and throat (ENT) surgery. Dr. Neel had been trained and practiced ENT all over the world. He had worked and lived from Europe to the continent of Africa before returning to Lucedale. Dr. Neel provided an expert level of ENT and plastic surgery to George County patients until 2008.

As advancements were made in the field of obstetrics and gynecology, GCH recruited and hired its first board-certified obstetrician gynecologist (OB/GYN), Dr. Kornstein, in 1996.

Dr. Denise Teasley, also an OB/GYN, arrived in 1998 to complete the OB/GYN program that had been started. Dr. Teasley set the standard for excellence in women's healthcare that continues to this day.

The family-medicine and general-practice doctors of GCH had delivered babies and provided women's healthcare from the beginning. But this program ushered in the modern era of women's health.

The advancements in healthcare in the first fifty years of GCH are too many to list. Worth mentioning, however, is the excellent level of surgical healthcare that was provided to the citizens of George County and the surrounding area, during the time before all the modern equipment and medications became available.

George County (now Regional) Hospital continues to offer the citizens of our area the most excellent and advanced surgical care available. These surgical specialties include: general surgery, OB/GYN, orthopedic, ENT, ophthalmology, and invasive radiology.

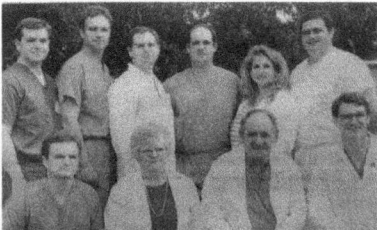

Front L-R: Heath Scott, MD, Laverne Scott, RN, Keith Scott, CRNA, Rhett Scott, CRNA

Back L-R: Paul Scott, MD, Mark Scott, RN, Seth Scott, MD, Derrick Scott, CRNA, Tara Mallett, DO, Brian Scott, RN

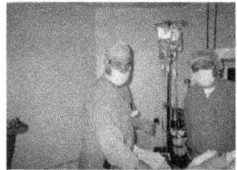

Derrick Scott

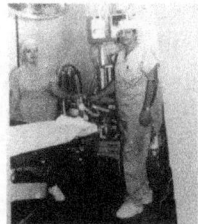

Rosemary Pankratz and Keith Scott

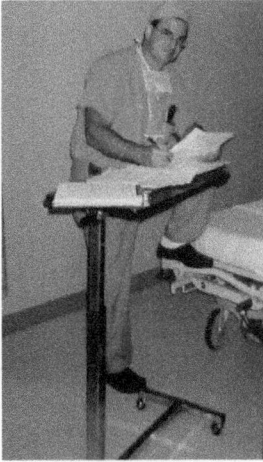

Rhett Scott

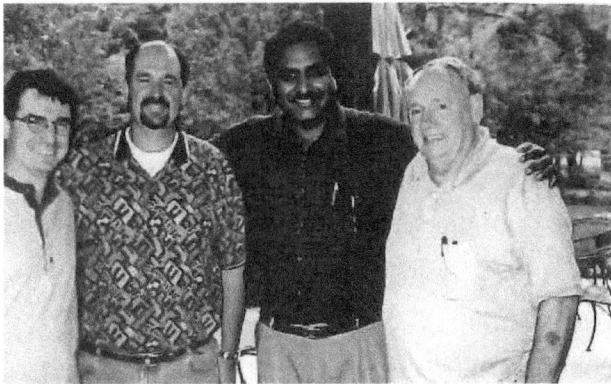

l-r: Rhett Scott, Derrick Scott, Dr. Suresh, Keith Scott

Surgeons

1950-2000

Dr. Raymond Benson (1950-1955)

Dr. Littleton (Lit) Eubanks (1950-1977)

Dr. Victor Landry (1953-1994)

Dr. Daniel Gonzalez (1960-1996)

Dr. Thompson (1964-1975) Came from Moss Point weekly

Dr. Herbert Kinsey (1975-1980)

Dr. Orndorff (10/1978-8/1979)

Dr. Dewey Lane (1964-1975) Came from Pascagoula weekly

Dr. Tan (10/1981-10/1982)

Dr. Robinson (1988)

Dr. Suresh Chintamaneni (1988-1997)

Dr. Rufus Neel (1992-2009)

Dr. Kornstein (1996-1998)

Dr. Martin Howard (2000)

Dr. Denise Teasley (1998-2008)

Dr. Weiss (1/1998-5/1998)

Dr. Fawaz (8/8/1999-8/31/1999)

Dr. David Crump (4/2000-7/2018)

Dr. Bobby Burn (3/2000-present)

Some of the other consulting physicians/surgeons through the years: Dr. James Harrison, Dr. Stephen Cope, Dr. Andy McLeod, Dr. Joseph McGowin III, Dr. Christopher Wiggins, Dr. Robert McGinley

Anesthesia Department:

First 50 Years

By Derrick Scott

As most people know, surgery would not be possible without anesthesia. Mrs. Grace Chalin, RN and Keith Scott, CRNA established the first full-time 24-hour-per-day anesthesia department at George County Hospital.

When Mr. Scott started in 1960, anesthesia was a relatively new art. Nurse anesthesia had only been around since 1930. Anesthesia gases in the 1960s were very explosive and operating room fires were a real concern. Even static electricity could cause a gas to ignite and result in explosion.

Mr. Scott was in solo practice 24 hours a day, 7 days a week. The only time he ever left town was for two weeks in the summer with his family for vacation. An out-of-town anesthetist would come stay at his house while he, his wife and their eight children traveled, usually visiting relatives in other states.

He continued this solo practice until 1974, when Ms. Rosemary Pankratz, CRNA, and her family moved to town. When he went on call every other week, it was "just like being on vacation". Ms. Pankratz practiced anesthesia from 1974 to 1993.

Mr. Scott's wife, Lavern Howell Scott, RN, worked as an operating room circulating nurse alongside him for 33 years.

This hospital is in my memory as far back as I can remember. It has been a source of income and influence on my entire family. Some of my earliest memories are of being handed over to my grandmother on her front porch by my parents on their way for emergency surgery.

Of the children of Keith and Laverne Scott, all eight worked at the hospital in some capacity:

1. Derrick Scott, CRNA

2. Rhett Scott, CRNA

3. Mark Scott, RN Director of Nursing

4. Dr. Tara Mallette, Pediatrician

5. Dr. Seth Scott, Family Medicine

6. Brian Scott, RN, staff nurse

7. Dr. Paul Scott, Urologist

8. Dr. Heath Scott, worked summers at the hospital while in medical school. He now practices Family Medicine in Yazoo City, MS.

While providing anesthesia, Keith Scott also served as interim administrator on two occasions. We still strive to carry on the tradition of hard work and care that he instilled in us.

Nursing

Directors of Nursing

1. INEZ HARMAN
2. ANNIS SHAW
3. BONNIE PAYNE
4. KAREN HOWELL
5. LAVERNE SCOTT
6. LENA WOZENCRAFT
7. ANITA LOTT (INTERIM)
8. PAT SHAW
9. CHRISTINE DAVIS
10. KATHRYN COOLEY
11. FREIDA DAVIS PIERCE
12. LINDA HOLLAND
13. MARK SCOTT

Nursing

By Patricia Howell, RN

Beginning in 1975

During nursing school we were required to do a clinical rotation at George County Hospital. We wore nursing caps then and our hair could not touch our collar. Shoes were to be pristine and no nail polish or jewelry except a wedding ring could be worn.

Annis Shaw, RN was the Director of Nursing and captain of a tightly run ship. She had a stern demeanor but she was very compassionate and obviously loved nursing. She was the epitome of what we deemed the perfect nurse. Tall, stately and starched, she marched the halls of "first desk" and "second desk", seeing all the patients and often rounding with the doctors. She was very involved with patient care in addition to all of her administrative duties.

After graduation from LPN school, Mrs. Shaw gave me my first nursing job in 1976. She hired Diane Miller, also fresh out of school, at the same time. We soon began taking classes along with Christine Davis to become RNs. The hospital gave me an educational allotment for continuing education in exchange for post graduate service. This allowed me to avoid student loans and was very much appreciated.

We kept a full house, the rooms were semi private, but you would have a private room if you had an illness that was communicable. Females shared rooms, males shared rooms and there was a curtain that could be pulled across in the middle for privacy or to keep the peace. We often kept patients up to 2 weeks or even longer, so there were times when we would be required to put patients in the hall with folding screens around them for privacy. The hospital payment system was very different then. Insurance companies and Medicare did not dictate length of stay and what tests were covered. All decisions regarding care were at the discretion of the patients' physician.

The nursing schedule was posted on a large piece of white board on the wall in the dining hall. The assignments for patient care or medication administration were given. In 1976 we had a drug room at the end of hall midway between desk one and two. The medication orders were taken from the chart by the unit clerk and written on cards of varying color depending on route of administration and checked off by a nurse for accuracy. These cards were labeled with the patient's name, room number, medication and dose as well as timing. These were put in order on a tray that held small paper or plastic cups and prepared by the LPN assigned to meds from the stock bottles in the drug room. A few years later the facility purchased a machine that dispensed the patient's medications in small plastic boxes. These boxes were prefilled by the nurse in charge of the drug room, Mrs. Ruth Stonecypher.

There were 3 shifts then. 7am-3pm, 3pm-11pm, and 11pm-7am. You could differentiate the shift charting by the color of ink used. Blue for days, green for evenings and red for nights. The shifts had some permanent nurses and aides but some floated among all the shifts and quite frequently you were asked to "volunteer" to pull a double if someone called in and no coverage could be found. We had some great nurse aides, Jake Rounsville, Gladys Mercer, Marcelle Leggett, Ms. Mcleod , "Patterson", and Jill Davis just to name a few. There were so many great nurses in those decades, I can't recall all their names so I won't try for fear of leaving someone out, but they all played a role in making our hospital a great place to work and to receive medical care. The work was hard, but there was a camaraderie among the staff that made the work very enjoyable.

We had patients in traction, under oxygen tents, and performed a variety of surgeries. There were 2 semi private rooms for obstetrics. Patient care involved a bath every day for everyone, shaves for the men, ambulating patients, IPPB treatments and percussive therapy (usually handled by Joyce Cochran, our unofficial respiratory therapist, gospel singer and coffee barista). We gave a lot of enemas in those days, a literal smorgasbord of enema types: soap suds enemas, tepid water enemas, fleets enemas, milk and molasses enemas, and one of Dr. Shaw's frequent orders, a 4H enema (high, hot, heck of a lot and hold it). We even gave enemas in the emergency room to infants and toddlers to reduce fever.

There were dressings to be changed, charts to check, orders to take off, admissions to take care of, and lights to answer. You never walked by a light above the door without going in. At bedtime (9pm), an aide brought a juice cart around and offered some to each patient allowed to have it, along with some crackers or melba toast. We also offered our patients a back rub and comfort measures at that time.

Dr. Whites and Dr. Shaw made formal rounds twice daily and popped in quite frequently at all hours of the day and night to check on patients, add orders or follow up on tests. They also covered the emergency room at night alternately so they both pretty much lived at the hospital. Dr. Landry and Dr. Gonzalez also worked at the hospital during that time and these 2 performed surgery as well as both having a private practice in town. They covered call for each other. Dr. Landry was a very snappy dresser in his polyester leisure suits (cutting edge fashion in those days) and he was very vocal in his displeasure when a newly hired young physician wore jeans to make rounds. I can still hear, in his gravelly, Louisiana accent, "it's juusst nawt professional!".

There was no ICU. Cardiac patients were kept in room 141. We had a very large cardiac monitor and crash cart combination on wheels that we connected to the patient.

A nurse was assigned to sit with that single patient all shift, providing private duty and close cardiac monitoring. Of course, only the nurses who had attended and passed a 3 week long cardiac course at Mobile Infirmary could be assigned to these acutely ill patients. There were no visiting cardiologists, our doctors took care of every type patient.

Many of our nurses were flexible and cross trained to work multiple departments. If you worked the emergency room(s), we had 2, then you also had to ride the ambulance when there was a call for one or if there was a transfer from the hall to another facility. Then one of the nurses from desk one had to be pulled to cover the emergency room. The emergency room nurse also had to go to the obstetrical suite if a delivery came in. If the ER nurse went to labor and delivery, a nurse from the hall was moved to the emergency room to cover for her. The ER nurses were cross trained to set up the delivery room and assist with the delivery as well as care for the newborn. The nursery was across from the nurse station at desk 2 and circumcisions were also performed there. I remember once a nurse asked Dr. Shaw jokingly what he was doing to make that baby cry and he responded, "I'm sharpening his pencil so he can make his mark". Dr. Shaw always had a joke to tell you.

Ancillary staff were also cross trained to perform multiple duties. Clyde Blackston worked as a male attendant but was also called upon to ride on the ambulance to help during emergencies and transfers. He would help out in the kitchen or housekeeping too if the need arose. J.C. Jack also performed these duties and at Christmas would dress in a Santa suit and visit all the patients spreading good cheer. George Parker was one of the few male nurses here at that time and was well loved by both patients and employees. Because he was male, he was often mistakenly called Dr. Parker by the patients.

Policies and procedures were very different then, there was no HIPAA. The hospital census was released readily and the patient list was called out over the airwaves every day by our local radio station, WRBE. We never worried about giving condition reports to anyone who asked about a patient. There were times that a particular physician would not allow us to tell a patient their diagnosis. "You will have to discuss that with your doctor", we were told to say if they asked. Smoking was very common and allowed in designated areas of the hospital. Ash trays were in every room.

Our IV fluids were contained in one liter glass bottles. We used syringe disposal containers with an attachment that cut the needle off to prevent reuse. We washed our hands pre and post procedure, but didn't wear gloves to give injections or draw blood. Bloodborne pathogens were not in the headlines then and HIV was unheard of.

In the event of dehydration in toddlers and no venous access, the physician would order clysis. The RN would insert needles into the subcutaneous tissue of the thigh bilaterally, connect a "Y" tubing, and allow fluids to infuse into alternate thighs. This method was highly successful in rehydration. Dr. Tipton at times would order turpentine stupes for abdominal distention. A turpentine concoction was applied topically to the abdomen, followed by the repeated application of warm moist towels. For active upper gi bleeding, we inserted a nasogastric tube and instilled iced normal saline with Levophed added. We didn't perform epidurals so our obstetrical patients received a pudendal block just before delivery. Even the rate, ratio and medications administered during CPR were different then.

Medicine and treatments as well as the method of delivery have changed so much since those years. The concepts that govern the day to day operations of the hospital environment have changed. The culture has changed. The appearance of the structure has changed. We have so much more available. Modes and modalities that were only available at distant facilities back then, are readily accessible now right here in our hometown. Thanks to an initial small group of citizens who had a vision, the hard work and planning of vested individuals as well as the knowledge and skill of professionals, both medical and non-medical, we have a facility that continues to thrive and provide exceptional medical care for George County and surrounding areas.

Second Graduating LPN Class

Seated L-R: Christine Davis, Lydia Beard, Barbara Emfinger

Standing L-R: Frieda Davis (Instructor), Charlene Harless, Shirley Leggett, Barbara Mc-Lendon, Stephenia Breland, Marie Campbell, Harlene Howell

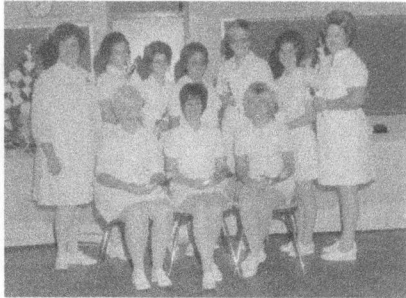

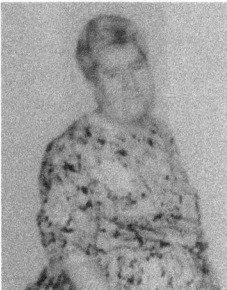

Emma Fallon

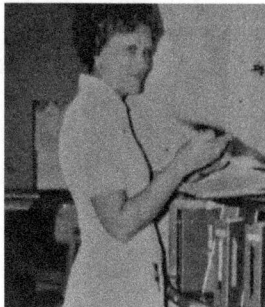

Pat Taylor Shaw

Nursing

By Christine Davis: 1974-1989

I began working at George County Hospital in 1974 as a licensed practical nurse (LPN). I was a 7-3 floor nurse who did many jobs. The main one was administering medications to the patients.

When patients were admitted to a room on the floor, and orders received from the admitting physician, the ward clerk would transcribe the orders to the patient's chart. The orders for meds were placed at the top of the charts which contained multiple carbon copies. These orders contained the name of the meds, the dosage, and the time to be given. They were then placed on med cards, which were color coded. Blue was for IV meds, yellow for IM meds, and white was for PO meds. The med cards included patient's name, room number, name of medication, and times to be given.

After physician's orders were checked by a registered nurse (RN) or LPN and orders were signed off, the cards were given to the "med nurse". She then took the med cards to the room where medications were kept. The drug room was kept stocked with all the meds physicians ordered. There she would pour up meds from large multidose bottles into med cups. The cups were placed into a tray which held many cups. These were the meds to be given at 9 a.m. The meds were given the same at each dose.

They were then taken to the patient's room, where arm bands on patients were checked to make sure medications were given to the correct patient. Then, after all the meds were given, the nurse would return to the nurses' station and place her initials in the top the nurse's notes and sign her name and initials at the bottom of nurses' notes where nurses signed and placed their initials.

All control drugs were kept in a double-locked cabinet at the nurses' station. They were counted by the off-going and oncoming med nurses or RN at the beginning and end of each shift. When count was complete and all drugs accounted for, each nurse who counts would sign the drug sheet.

Mrs. Ruth Stonecypher, LPN, would keep drugs replaced after they were checked by the registered pharmacist. These pharmacists used were local drug store pharmacisits.

At the second nurses' station, there was a room on the hall that housed a large autoclave. It was used to autoclave the metal bed pans, urinals, and other metal equipment used by patients. At this time, these objects were not disposable. This was done by the nurses on duty. As a floor nurse, you would rotate from Nurse Station One and Nurse Station Two to the Emergency Department and Labor and Delivery if needed.

At Nurse Station One, there was a patient room next to it designated as a pediatric room. It contained a baby bed, cot, straight chairs, and rocking chairs.

Before we had an intensive care unit/cardiac care unit (ICU/CCU), the cardiac patients were admitted to Room #141, across from Nurse Station One. The nurses who worked in this room had received a 120-hour course at Mobile Infirmary pertaining to cardiac patients.

After the four-bed ICU/CCU opened, many of the RNs received their advanced cardiac life support (ACLS) certificated. This course took three days to complete. By 1987, there were twelve RNs who had completed the course. These nurses were recognized by the administrator, Mr. Rupert Ingram. He also recognized Mrs. Annis Shaw, RN for fifty two years of service. She had been at George County for twenty years.

After working 3-11 on the floor, I was transferred to the Emergency Department (ED). During this time, if a call came in for an ambulance, the ED nurse would go with the driver and a male attendant on the ambulance. The ED would be covered by a nurse from the floor until the ambulance returned.

Sometimes, the patient coming to the ED in the ambulance would be transferred to an outlying hospital. The ED nurse, an LPN, would go on transfers unless the physician requested that an RN go.

At this time, there were two ED rooms located in the back of the hospital where the ambulances were located. As you came up the ramp at the back, you came into the hospital. There was a registration desk as you came through the door and next to that area was a waiting room for patients who were waiting to be seen by the physician.

The ED rooms were on each side of the hall. Room One was on the right which housed an exam table for patients to be examined. This exam table also could be used as an exam table to do proctoscopes which the doctors would use sometimes.

Later on, two more ED rooms were added to the back of ED Two. These were across from the entrance to the dining room.

During my time in the ED, if any obstetrical (OB) patient stating she was in labor came to the emergency department, the RN from Nurse Station One was notified. She would come to the ED and find out if the patient was having contractions and how long she had been having them. She would examine the patient to see if she was in active labor. Then she would notify the physician.

If orders were given to put the patient in a labor room and monitor patient, she was placed on fetal monitor. This allowed the nurse to check how far apart her contractions were, if the baby was having any problems with labor, if labor was progressing and if baby was showing signs of deceleration of its heartbeat during contractions. If mother was dilated far enough, the physician may apply a scalp monitor to the baby. That monitor would be removed at the time of delivery.

After the baby's delivery and APGAR score, baby would be transferred to the newborn nursery located across the hall from Nurse Station Two. It had glass windows on two sides. One side faced the nurses' station. The other side faced the hall where new mothers were housed.

Sometimes, if an OB patient stayed in labor for a long period and no progression was noted, the physician may decide the patient needed a cesarean section (C-section). The physician would notify a surgeon and the C section would be done. After the baby was delivered and APGAR scores done, the baby was taken to the newborn nursery and the mother was taken to the recovery room until she awoke. Then, she was transferred to the OB rooms on the floor.

Sometimes, if babies were having trouble in the nursery, they may be transferred to Mobile Infirmary which had a neonatal ICU. Their staff would come to George County in their ambulance which was well equipped for this purpose. They would also bring the nurses who work in the Neonatal unit.

In 1978, I began working on getting my RN degree. I took night classes at the vocational center for a year to get as many classes as possible. In 1979, I entered the RN program at Jackson County Junior College to begin studying for an associate's degree. In nursing, all my classes were in the morning hours. After classes, I worked the 3-11 shift at George County Hospital, in ICU or on the floor.

I received my diploma in May 1981. I received my RN license in May of 1982. In the latter part of 1982 or early part of 1983, I was appointed to the position of director of nursing (DON). There were many changes going on at the hospital. We were joined by Mobile Infirmary.

Several workers took EMT courses because they were sometimes asked to ride in the ambulance with patients. Several were registered EMT, ambulance. At this time, I started as a part-time ambulance driver.

While serving as DON, one thing I really wanted to happen was to allow OB fathers to participate in the labor and delivery of their babies. There were a lot who were grateful for this opportunity. There was only one father who felt faint and had to sit down against the wall.

When the hospital opened in 1950, the newborn nursery was located at Nurse Station One, so were the OB rooms. Across from the nurses' station were the OB rooms and beside the station was the newborn nursery. This remained until sometime after 1960.

By 1966, the newborn nursery and OB rooms were located at Nurse Station Two. On May 23, 1966, the OB rooms and newborn nursery were integrated. The integration went smoothly without any incident.

Nursing

By Dianne Miller, RN

My introduction to the hospital environment began in 1975 when I entered George County Hospital as a fledgling nursing student. With several weeks of classroom study, and weeks of clinical training at the local nursing home under our belts, we arrived on the hospital threshold, starched and polished under the tutelage of our instructors, Freida Davis, RN and Mary Ann Byrd, RN.

We had very strict instructions regarding patient care and assessment techniques. We were given in depth education regarding aseptic technique, injection administration, foley catheter insertion, enema administration, and dressing changes. Of course, all procedures had to be done under the eagle eye of one of our instructors. There were many patients in the hospital in those days so there was ample opportunity to get "signed off" on your procedures and then you could perform them independently.

Those 12 months passed by quickly and upon graduation, I was hired by the hospital. Annis Shaw, RN was the Director of Nursing and she hired several of the graduates in my class. More nurses were required in those days because there were 3 eight-hour shifts to cover. The usual staffing pattern included a Registered Nurse for each of the 2 nursing stations (desk 1 and 2), 2-3 LPNs for patient care, treatments or medication administration and 2-3 nurse aides for patient care. The aides were not certified in those days. They were trained on the job. We usually had one male attendant per shift to assist with male patients and lifting large patients. There was usually an LPN assigned to the emergency room too. She floated to OB, rode the ambulance and assisted at desk 1 or recovery, if no patients were in the emergency room.

The departments were not as structured in the 70's. We just helped all over the hospital where there was a need. The doctors made rounds twice daily. Early am and again after lunch. We tried to be prepared for them by having all the charts loaded in wheeled carts. We kept prescription pads and pens readily available for them and often wrote the orders in the chart as the doctor dictated them to us. There was no automation, lots of handwritten pages, forms, and paper reports to put on the chart. The unit secretary was a valued team member. I was privileged to work with a lot of them.

The actual charts in the 70's were made of metal, flat with allergy stickers or other memos of importance stuck on front. They were kept in a rack connected to the desk where the nurse charted, the unit clerk sat and the phone was located. In the 80's we advanced to ringed binder charts with dividers that were housed in a carousel at the desk. The orders, lab requests, and x-ray requests were all produced with carbon copies. Each copy had a designated destination. With the longer patient stays the chart would become quite thick and it would be "reduced" with the older information housed in another binder but accessible until discharge. The total discharge chart may be 4-8 inches thick.

All patients were considered "inpatients" then and having procedures done "outpatient" was not a priority. Cardiac patients with fresh MI's may be kept as long as 3 weeks to recover. During high census times patients were kept in the hallway with privacy screens and in the lobby of the physical therapy department located at the end of the hall adjacent to desk 2. On rare occasions we would add a third bed to a room to accommodate the influx of patients.

The nursery was across from desk 2 and the babies stayed in there except for brief visits with the mothers. We had 4 obstetrical beds, 2 in each room. Circumcisions were performed in the anteroom of the nursery. Papoose boards were used to immobilize the infant. The nursery was attended by a nurse aide and the RN in charge at desk 2 was responsible for infant care. I remember 2 older aides that worked in the nursery were Mrs. Sanderson and Mrs. Collins. They could always be seen through the plate glass window, rocking a baby.

The semiprivate arrangement made for some interesting connections and conversations. Some amiable, some not. Privacy was certainly not a really high priority then. A curtain could be pulled for visual privacy but conversations were not private and the patients shared a telephone situated between the beds.

We had many surgery patients because Dr. Landry, Dr. Gonzalez and Dr. Kinsey performed all types of surgery. We used portable Gumco suction machines for continuous gastric suction, portable suction machines for naso-oropharyngeal suction, portable diathermy machines, and lymphedema pumps. A lot of our nursing care was hard physical labor. Moving and operating the various machines, emptying, measuring outputs and cleaning at each shift change. Lifting patients manually as there were no Hoyer lifts. Applying traction with varying amounts of weight was another task we often performed.

There was no ICU in the mid-seventies so when we had a cardiac or respiratory arrest on the hall, a code 100 was called over the intercom and anyone available responded. There was no code team. Of course, there was another patient in the room that had to be evacuated, calmed and settled somewhere. A nurse would grab the huge crash cart with a monitor and defibrillator on top and push as quickly as possible to the room. Often a portable x-ray machine would be brought. The portable EKG machine was brought. Someone would call the doctor if he wasn't already in the hospital. Someone from lab would respond because they would certainly require bloodwork. It was not uncommon to have a student nurse or two trapped in the corner. Several nurses would be there to perform CPR, administer meds, and/or document events. The small room would be filled to capacity.

We took care of patients of all ages. We had 2 rooms on the 100 hall that had murals painted in them and these were the pediatric rooms. I remember once there was a very sick child in one of those rooms. He had laryngeotracheobronchitis and was under an oxygen tent. We had a lot of peds with tents then. Dr. Tipton stayed all night and paced the halls to be available for that child.

Our doctors were very "hands on" in the treatment of their patients and it was never surprising to go into a room on your hourly rounds and find the doctor in there at any time of the day or night. The doctor's wives must have been very generous and understanding because it seemed the doctors essentially lived at the office and the hospital.

Shortly after I came to work at the hospital, I realized I had found my niche and wanted to return to school and obtain my Registered Nurse degree. I convinced my friend and coworker Pat Davis to do the same. She had attended LPN training with me and we worked well together. We began in the late 70's and finished in the early 80's. During this time the Director of Nursing arranged our schedule so we could work all weekend and remain full time at the hospital. After I got my Registered Nursing license, I was immediately promoted to day shift supervisor.

I've worked since then in various administrative roles. I was interim Director of Nurses for a brief period in the eighties. I gained a wealth of experience during my tenure in those decades because we provided care for all types of illness. We progressed as procedures, techniques and knowledge evolved. I think flexibility and versatility are essential traits necessary to succeed as a nurse in a small hospital. After 17 years of full-time nursing in a supervisory role, I decided to decrease my work schedule to a prn basis. I took a short hiatus, became very bored and decided to return full time to the hospital a year or so prior to Y2K. It was like I had returned home. I've had the privilege to work with some of the best doctors, nurses, aides and unit secretaries on the planet. I've been very blessed.

Nursing

Christine Stevens Weiland RN, MSN

1974-1984

My career in Nursing grew deep from within the halls of George County Hospital.

In 1974, I began my career in nursing while a Senior at George County High School in the Occupational Health Program. Ms. Georgia Rouse RN was the first nursing instructor to walk me & my dear friend Belva Anderson Hayden down the halls of George County Hospital. Lord, had we only known where that walk would take us!

There we were introduced to the basics of nursing, the activities of daily living, feeding, bathing & ambulation. It's been almost 50 years but some things have not changed. While assisting with breakfast trays & the feeding of patients I can still hear the sound of the cart which was carrying the patient charts & being pushed down the halls by Dr. Whites, Dr. Shaw, and Dr. Tipton. Ms. Annis Shaw, RN who was the Director of Nursing would always follow them down the hall. She reminded me of Bambi's father entering the forest. You always knew when the Prince of the forest arrived. She carried such a presence of respect & admiration. Later you would see Dr. Landry & Dr. Gonzalez make rounds. As a young frightened student, I always knew to quietly scurry from their sight. Hours later after the charts had been reviewed & doctor orders "taken off" by Ms. Helen Allen, RN, I would see her walk down the halls with her IV tray, one patient after the other, she would start everyone's IV's & give all the IV meds. I remember the nursing aides Joyce Cochran & Marcella Leggett smiling & singing in the halls. Those were the first days I began to detect the smell of sickness, the look of death upon the face & the grimacing of agonizing pain.

At 1130 each morning, we would leave the halls of George County Hospital & reload onto the yellow school bus to return to GCHS for afternoon classes. Many days, Belva & I would see classmates who had skipped the clinical rotation at the hospital sneak onto the bus to return as if they had been with us at the hospital. They would laugh & talk of their fun times using LSD in some old house nearby while we had been learning how to care for sick patients all morning. Needless to say they never furthered their education in nursing. Belva & I are still nurses today.

After graduating from George County High School in 1975 I entered the Licensed Practical Nursing Program at MGCCC. Once again in August, I returned to the halls of George County Hospital. This time Belva wasn't with me but Diane Miller was. Once again I would see the same doctors making rounds, writing orders then Ms. Allen taking all the orders off, checking & rechecking her IV orders. Ms Allen was always there, always on duty, always working. I never saw her eat, I never saw her sit down. As an LPN student I worked with the medicine nurse mostly. I remember giving my first suppository. I remember asking what was route 1 as the order was written ....insert RT1. I can still see the face & hear the laugh of my nursing instructor, Freida Davis, RN as she told me it meant to insert it rectally. I still feel the embarrassment of my" Route 1" question. I love how Ms. Freida could teach & laugh with us but not laugh at us. I can still see her beautiful face laughing in the halls of George County Hospital way back in the Seventies. I can still see her face over me when I was "coming back around" after fainting all 12 times.

She never once told me I would never make it as a nurse because I fainted with every new sight & smell of nursing procedures. To her I owe my first nursing's license.

In Sept. 1976, I was hired as a new LPN graduate at George County Hospital by Ms. Shaw, Director of Nursing. She was a true icon of George County Hospital during the days when nurses were starched stiff in white dresses & stiff caps. Although she never said it, you automatically knew she demanded excellent nursing care. Versatility & multitasking of nursing duties nor floating were words of the Seventies. Very simplistically, you knew you went to work where ever you were told to go & figured out what to do the best you could. I would be assigned to work in the pharmacy to assist Ms. Ruth Stonecypher many days, as well as work as the ambulance nurse if a call came in. Ms. Stonecypher was an LPN who operated the pharmacy with a pharmacist signing off on the work she & I would complete. I believe she was one of George County Hospital's finest!! During my years of working with her I was molded thru her integrity & dedication to the profession of nursing as well as her love for George County Hospital & her community.

In 1978, I completed the EMT-A certification & began working as an Ambulance Nurse & in the Emergency room. During the seventies, the Emergency Room had 2 Exam rooms & would only be staffed when a patient arrived. If the switchboard received a call requesting an ambulance, an ambulance driver would be called at home to come to the hospital, pick up the ambulance nurse & go provide care for the emergency patient. A doctor would be on call so when a patient arrived at the hospital with an emergency, a nurse would be sent from the floor to the ER to assess the patient & determine if a doctor needed to be called. If so, then the doctor would come from home to care for the emergency patient. The hours I worked as an ambulance nurse at George County Hospital was my most influential experience in the development of my nursing knowledge

& skills & path of specialization in my 45 years of nursing. I remember after we had completed the care on a traumatic case," Ole Doctor Tip" as we knew him, told me "You need to go to Gulfport, this place is too small for you". I didn't have a clue what he meant but later I did just as he recommended. This year makes 35 years of nursing for me in Gulfport. Today, his son works down the hall from me. Even he has never heard my story of what prompted me to move from George County & go work in Gulfport.

Nearly 50 years later I can only imagine how the faces of Diane Miller & Belva Hayden must appear still going down the halls of George County Hospital. I assume the students of 2020 will refer to them as I referred to Ms. Shaw & Ms. Allen. In my mind, they are now the icons of George County Hospital.

George County Hospital has always been where my heart of nursing lives. The "People" of the Seventies are engrained in my Memories from the Halls of George County Hospital.

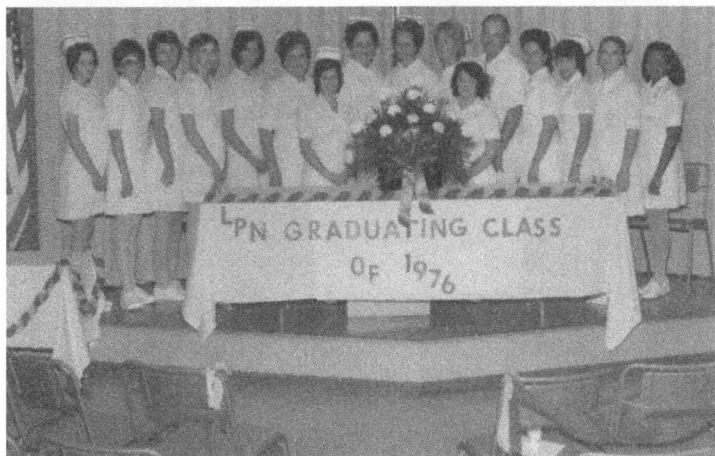

L-R: Christine Stevens Weiland, Dianne Miller, Shannon Roberts, Pat Davis Howell, Lisa Faurot Freeman, Edna Hickman, Kathryn Cooley, unknown, unknown, Kathleen Dueitt, Regina Moody, George Parker, unknown, Sheila Kiser, Donna Courtney, unknown.

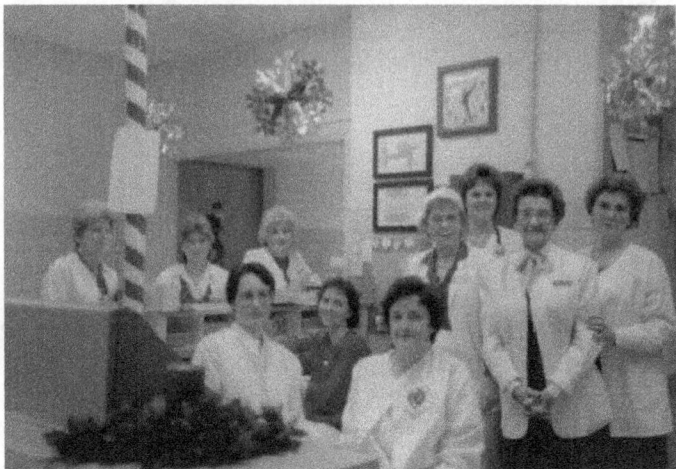

Seated L-R: Gloria Havard, Milta Bishop, Gwen Bobinger
Standing L-R: Annie Bell Strahan, Shirley Leggett, Shirley Thompson,
Christine Davis, Gail Tipton, Ms. McAlister, Doris Jean Eckhoff

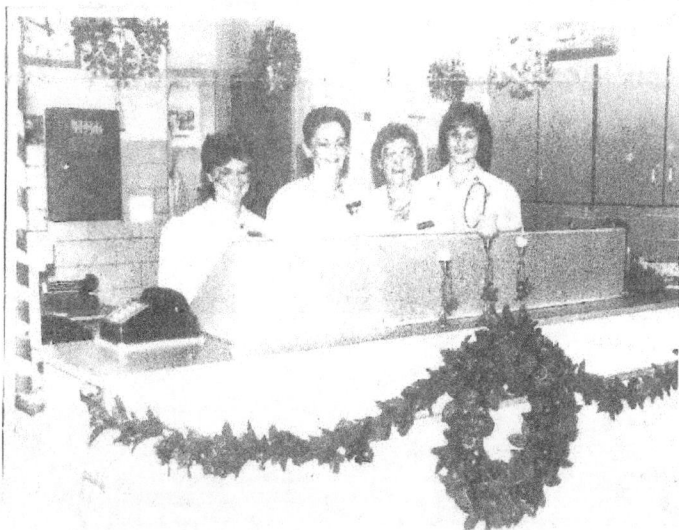

Second Place Winner...

THE NURSES STATION was the second place winner in the George County
Hospital's Christmas Decoration Contest. Pictured with some of their award winning
decorations are (from left to right) Shirley Leggett, Diane Miller, Christine Davis
(Director of Nurses) and Debbie Daughdrill.

Laboratory

by Joyce Horne Rutherford, MT (ASCP)

My history with the Lab at George County Hospital started in the summer of 1969. I had just finished my freshman year at Gulf Coast Community College (Perk) and needed some spending money for college life. Mr. Johnny Mills, who was Administrator at the time, was good enough to hire me. I was taking pre-medical courses and intended for Pharmacy to be my major as I had worked for Al Eubanks at Al's Pharmacy throughout high school. That summer job at the hospital changed my career path. I was intrigued by the laboratory procedures and the diagnostic capabilities and importance, and changed my major to Medical Technology.

When I started working, the staff included: Kathryn Nell Griffin, Gerald Evans, Doug Mixon, Becky Taylor, Nona Holloman and Lucille Lawrence. There was a lady that they often spoke of who had worked in the Lab and X-ray before my arrival by the name of "Mac" Havard.

Becky trained me to perform EKGs, which fell under Lab responsibilities at the time. The EKGs had to be carried to the bus station, which was also a gas station on Main Street owned by Mr. Sam Bristow. They had to be there before 11a.m. to travel by bus to Mobile to be read by cardiologists.

Then later, EKGs were transmitted by the "Data-phone", a device in which you placed the telephone receiver in a small box after placing electrodes in appropriate places on the patient. Sometimes, if it was an emergency, the cardiologist would dictate the report immediately over the phone when it was finished. I always dreaded this, nervous that I wouldn't get all the technical terms about inverted T-waves, ST segments, etc. accurate.

Once, the doctor came on the phone and said, "This man has had a heart attack!" There was a pause, so I asked, "Is that all?" He replied, "No, it's a bad one!" Of course, there were many other duties, filing, stocking, cleaning, making coffee and anything that the techs asked you to do. I learned a lot by watching and asking a lot of questions.

Eventually, they taught me how to draw blood which was a big help when I got to the clinical part of my studies. Dr. Faust, my Chemistry professor during my freshman and sophomore years in college, gave me special attention and privileges since I worked in a "Hospital Lab". Never mind that I was only a grunt!

I continued to work weekends, holidays and summers until I completed my degree in Medical Technology and worked every chance I got. I really enjoyed working there. We were a family! Everybody helped each other, no matter what your department.

I came to work as a tech in May 1973 and worked the evening shift. Sometimes, that shift wasn't very busy, so I helped out on the nursing floor or other areas, anything to stay busy. There were no computers or cell phones to occupy your time, not that I would have anyway. I was taught that when you worked for someone you worked your full shift. We also rotated taking call back in the early years, and even when you were at the hospital most of the night, you were expected back promptly for your shift the next day.

However, we did have some fun when all the chores were done, laughing at ourselves, playing tricks on each other, etc. Sometimes, we had to laugh in order to deal with the seriousness, sadness and often ugliness of the job.

We performed lab tests by hand when I first started working at GCH. There was no automation. We cooked blood sugars in Folin Wu tubes, poured them into a cuvette and read them on a Leitz photometer, to determine the glucose. We performed other chemistries (amylase, lipase, chloride, etc) in a similar manner. Blood cells were counted on a lined hemacytometer slide, observed under a microscope (usually a Leica). We measured hemoglobin using the photometer and centrifuged whole blood in tiny cylinders (capillary tubes) to measure hematocrit. This was called a "spun hematocrit" and was lined up and read on a chart.

One of the first instruments that I remember was an IL Flame photometer and I was scared to death of it because it had a small gas tank, and you had to actually light the flame to measure sodium (Na) and potassium (K). We eventually acquired a Beckman instrument that performed glucose and blood urea nitrogen (BUN). Carbon dioxide (CO_2) was measured in a glass contraption called a biuret, where mercury was poured into the top in a thermometer-like tube. The specimen was introduced at the bottom, and the contraption shook, forming the gas (CO_2) to be produced and measured in that tube. We kept mercury in a small bottle and "played" with it often. If any was spilled, you could easily roll it up into a ball and put it back in the bottle! Obviously, we didn't know about mercury poisoning back then! We had a Gamma Counter for measuring blood volumes.

The first semi-automated chemistry instrument that I remember at George County Hospital was the Clinicard made by IL (Instrumentation Laboratories). It used cartridges where you introduced a sample into the reagent cartridge, inserted it into the instrument, waited for a re-

action and recorded the results. The basic chemistry ana-
lytes were available through this system.

When I was in training at Singing River Hospital, the lab
there purchased a Technicon instrument that allowed us
to perform SMA-12 (Sequential Multiple Analyzer). This
was my first experience with automated chemistry instruments. Of course, as a student, I wasn't allowed to
actually TOUCH the instrument. It was very complicated
with thousands (it seemed like) tiny tubes intertwining
through the instrument. One of my favorite Techs there,
Patsy (who was a small person), seemed to always have
her head stuck up in that monstrosity working on it. The
SMA-12/60 allowed 12 determinations to be performed
on 60 specimens in one hour. Later on came the SMAC
(C stood for computer) and allowed 20-40 determinations
on 120 specimens in one hour.

At George County, the first automated chemistry instrument that I remember was made by Union Carbide (and
later became Baker Instruments) called the Centrifchem
purchased in May 1976. Other chemistry instruments that
came along were:

Abbott TDX in 1985, followed by the IMX. The Abbott
Spectrum in 1988 and the Abbott AxSYM shortly after.

Beckman instruments came next. Synchron CX5 at the
clinic lab and the CX7 at the hospital lab around 1995-96.
It became important for us to have compatible systems at
the clinic for back-up in case the instruments at the hospital went down. Our doctors had grown very dependent on
lab results, as they should! Having the instrumentation
in the clinic lab also allowed a better workflow for patient
care and offered a service most small labs did not provide.

Hematology instrumentation became automated in 1978
when we purchased our first Coulter Counter, the model
FN and then eventually the Model S. Coulter Electronics
was the name of the Hematology game for many years and
served us well. Then Abbott Laboratories got into the He-

matology business, and we purchased the CELL-DYN CC 780 in Aug 1987, followed by the KN models and then the K1000.

We used Leica microscopes and eventually Nikon. For coagulation, we used the tilt tube method in the beginning, and then the Fibrometer and an MLA system. We had various makes of centrifuges to prepare specimens, Drucker, Eppendorf and Beckman to name a few.

Microbiology was slow to be automated. We used sight and smell, simple tests and the microscope to read Gram stains. We used the API strip for bacterial identification and Kirby Bauer plates for sensitivities. This was all replaced or at least enhanced by the VITEK system around 1990. We continued to perform some tests by hand to aid in identification.

Blood bank was the last to be automated, probably due to its critical nature. An error in blood bank could cause death and we were all wary of trusting an automated system. We did compatibility testing (crossmatching) by hand. We performed what was called a 'major' and a 'minor' crossmatch, which was a double check on compatibility. We finally purchased a cell washer which saved a few steps.

We purchased a data management system (DataTrac) in 1988 which tied most of these systems together for concise, consolidated printed reports. This was eventually replaced by the Meditech information system, which linked all areas of the hospital by computer.

Over my forty-six years working at George County Hospital, I saw many changes, improvements in technology being the most significant. We progressed from offering around 20 tests in-house with a test volume of around 80 tests per day to offering around 100 tests in-house with a volume of around 500 tests per day, in addition to tests sent out to our reference lab.

Many employees contributed greatly to the success of our Department during the first fifty years. In addition to the ones mentioned before were Elouise Farish, Marilyn Hastings, Hilda Wilcutt, Paula Pankratz, Kathy Dale, Angie Kiser, Mary Kate Fairley, Marci Hayden, Gail Bond, Joann Baggett, Angela Burkett, Kay Pipkins, Sherry Beck, Robin Goff, Tammy Walley, Pat Berry, and others who were there for shorter periods of time, or came after the year 2000.

Consulting Pathologists were necessary and very important to the management of the Laboratory. They typically made monthly visits to review all laboratory results, tissue reports, blood utilization and to discuss and make recommendations to the Lab Director and Technologists. The Mississippi State Department of Health signed into law the Clinical Laboratory Act (CLIA) in 1988 for the oversight and certification of clinical Laboratory testing. This Act ensured quality testing and Pathologists were required to oversee the process. In the early years, we used Puckett Laboratories in Hattiesburg, MS for our Reference Lab and consulting Pathologists. Dr. Thomas F. Puckett and Dr. Robert S. Cooke were the most frequent Consulting Pathologists to our hospital and later, Dr. Thomas G. Puckett, when he took over the practice after his father's death.

But the thing I cherish most, especially in the earlier years, is what a family the employees were and how we truly cared for each other and our patients. We always wanted what was best for them and the hospital.

It was an honor and a pleasure to be a part of this organization for over forty years.

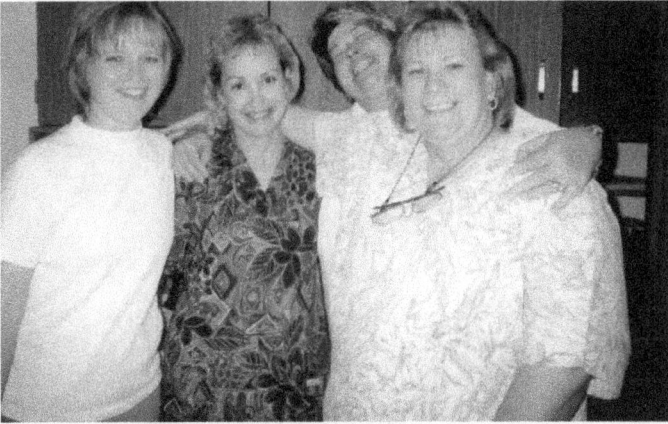

L-R: Joann Baggett, Mary Fairley, Betty (courier), Gail Bond

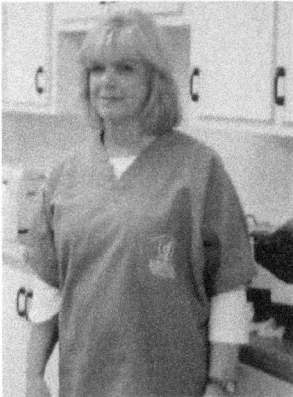

left: Joyce Rutherford

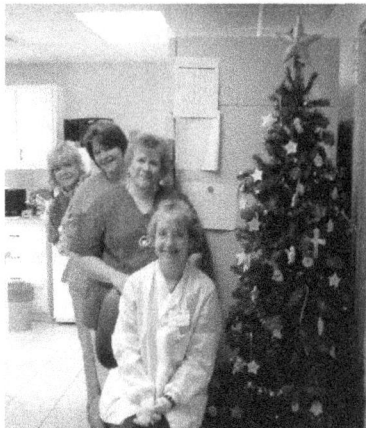

Front to Back: Mary Fairley; Gail Bond;
Laura Dueitt; Joyce Rutherford

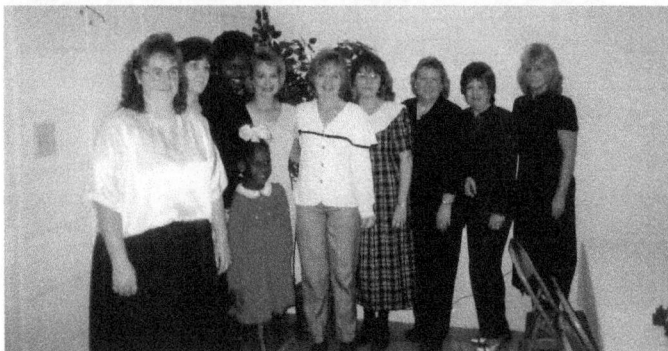

L-R: Tammy Walley, Paula Pankratz, Angela Burkett (daughter Ashley), Mary Fairley, Joann Baggett, Sherry Beck, Gail Bond, Elouise Farish, Joyce Rutherford

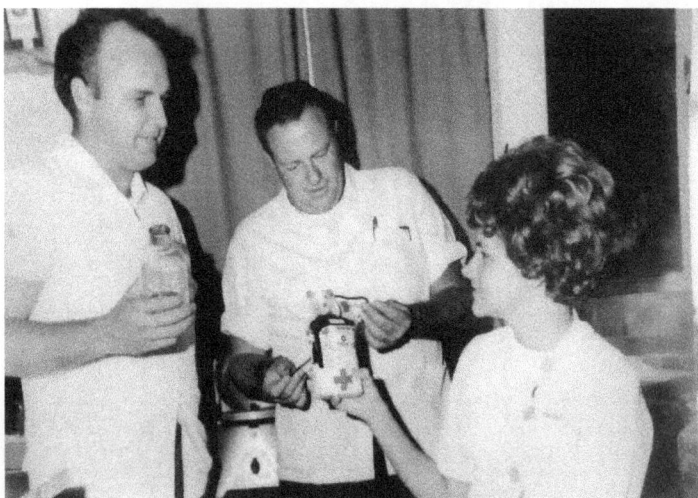

L-R: Gerald Evans, Doug Mixon, Kathryn Griffin

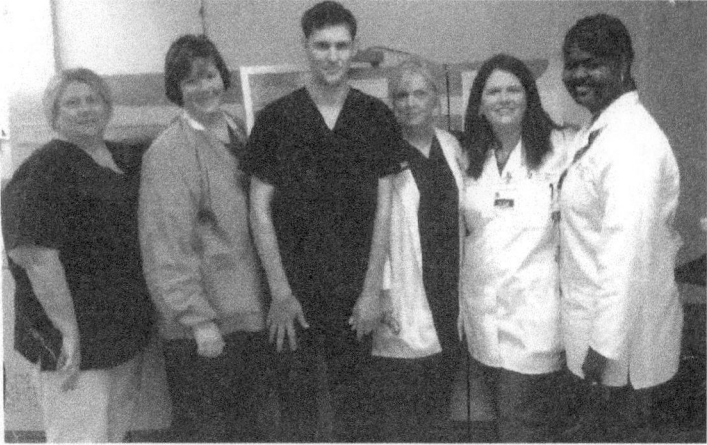

L-R: Gail Bond, Laura Dueitt, Jonathan Dixon, Joyce Rutherford,
Christie Morse, Angela Burkett

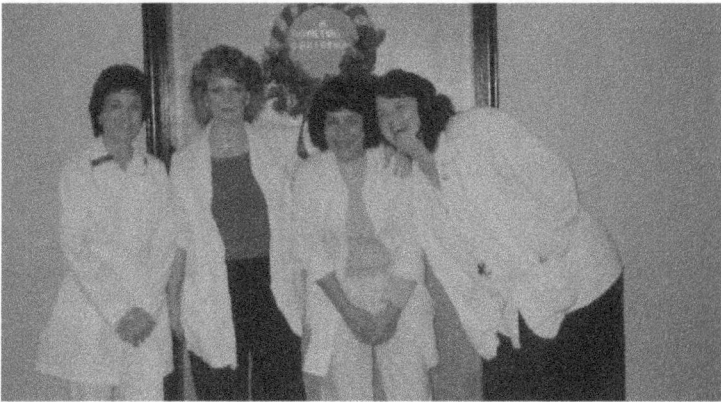

L-R: Elouise Bradley Farish, Joyce Rutherford, Kathy Dale, Angie Kiser

Radiology

By Christy Pope, RT(R), RDMS, RVT

Times were very different in the years preceding my arrival in the Radiology Department. A few of the names that I heard mention of were Vic Goodman, who was the Radiology Director for many years, Gerald Evans and Doug Mixon, who did X-ray and Lab, Rosa Bilbo, Dale Burnett, Patricia Maples, Debby Holland, Hazel Havard, Diane Touchstone, and David Draime. The Radiologists were Dr. Stroble, Dr. Sauls, Dr. Hale and Dr. Reikes.

X-rays were taken with a stationary unit and developed in dip tanks in a dark room. No Fluoroscopy, just still images. They were taken by bus to be dictated in Hattiesburg, MS.

I started working in the Radiology Department of George County Hospital in 1996. Sandy Sellers was the Director of Radiology at that time. He hired me to work part time on the weekends in X-ray while attending Ultrasound school full time. Upon completion of Ultrasound school I began working full time as a Sonographer. The staff consisted of Paul Martin; Assistant Director, Joyce Sellers and Jan Welford; Secretaries, Judy Hudson; Mammo and U/S, Jennifer Galle, Greg Havard, Harry Harrington, Keith Pierce; Technologist. The Radiologist was a group from Mobile. They came every weekday and left at lunch. The Administrator at this time was Paul Gardner.

During this time, all X-rays were developed in a dark room and run through a processor. There were no 'digital images'. We had film that had to be hung on a lighted view box. The Radiologist would dictate the report for the exam. We had an in-house transcriptionist that would type the report. One copy would go to the ordering physician, one copy to Medical Records, and one copy to the Radiology department. The copy for radiology would be put into the patient's folder along with their images and filed outside in a warehouse. Most evenings in the Radiology department consisted of filing all the reports in the folders and returning them outside to film storage. We sure hated rainy days because that meant you would stay wet all day having to pull folders from outside.

Our department was very compact to say the least. We had a Rad/Fluoro room where our fluoroscopy procedures were done. One Rad room which was shared with U/S. Mammography, Nuclear Medicine, and CT was in a trailer in front of hospital. Nuclear medicine shared a space with the inside file room. The Radiologist was in a very small 'closet' off of the Nuclear Medicine room. New Ultrasound equipment was purchased just as I was finishing U/S school and starting full time. The new equipment was put in a really small room adjacent to the secretary's office.

One thing that hasn't changed over the years is the warm family atmosphere. The employees truly care about each other and they have one common goal—To make a positive difference through excellent healthcare and service –every life, every moment, every day!

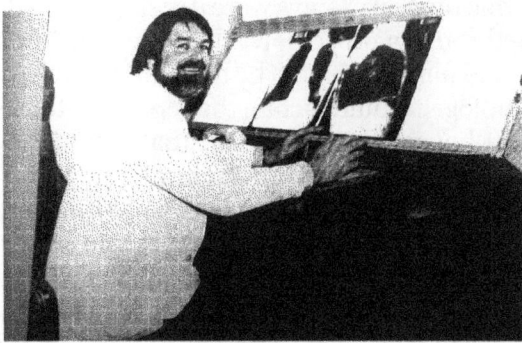

Victor Goodman

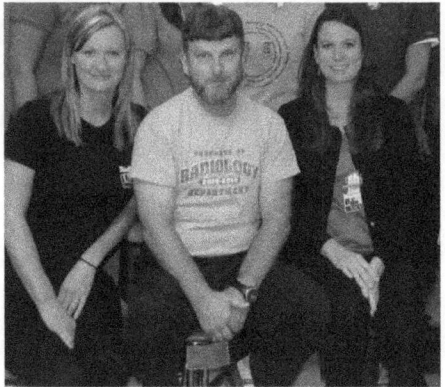

Christy Pope, Paul Martin, Jennifer Galle

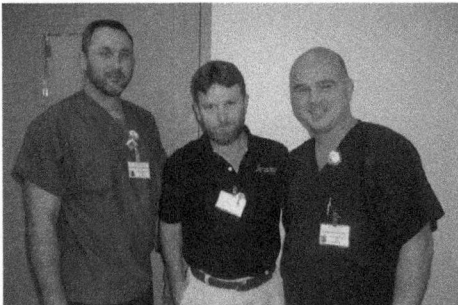

Delton McLain, Paul Martin, Jake McDaniel

Emergency Room

By Dr. Dayton Whites

When George County Hospital opened in 1950, there was a room 24ft x 24 ft near the rear entrance of the hospital which was the emergency room. Near the back door of the hospital was a buzzer button, which was used to summon a nurse from the nurses' desk. Patients presenting would use this method when appearing for emergency care.

Early on, this room was seldom used because all non-emergency patients were seen at the Doctor's office or at home. Seriously ill patients and severe accident patients were still seen at home and often transferred to Mobile by their family physician since there was no ambulance service. In 1961, The Medical Staff felt the emergency patients and other patients could receive better treatment in the emergency room than on home calls or in the physician's office.

Financial arrangements would be as follows: the ER would charge $1.50 per patient visit and the Medical Staff would charge $4.00 to come and check patients. At that time, office visits were $3.00and house calls were $5.00 plus 50 cents per mile, one way. Local physicians would see their own patients. The staff physicians would care for patients without a local doctor on a rotation basis.

The system worked well for many years. ER visits increased over the next several years. In the mid 1970's, the hospital administrator approached Dr. Tom Shaw and Dr.

Dayton Whites about weekend coverage for the ER. It was agreed upon that the two of them would cover the ER from 5:00 pm on Friday until 7:00 am on Monday. They would see all patients who came to the ER, and they would also cover all inpatients at the hospital.

The physician pay for the coverage would be $25 per hour. Also, the hospital would place a trailer behind the hospital as living quarters for the physician on call. This system worked well for the hospital and local physicians.

ER visits continued to rise during these years. The next move towards full-time ER physician coverage would be adding ER physicians for weeknight coverage. Administration contacted the University of South Alabama for help. It was decided that second and third-year USA Medical residents would cover the ER, not only on weekends but also weeknights, 7:00pm to 7:00am. This worked well and this system was used for about 10 years. Some of the notable ER physicians were:

Dr. Frank Martin

Dr. Frank Bunch

Dr. Richard Johnson

Dr. John Pavlov

Full time ER physician coverage at George County Hospital would come in the early 1990's. Dr. John Van Derwood and his wife, Dr. Karen Jimenez, along with other physicians would start 24 hour, 7 day a week coverage for the ER. In 1994 Dr. Joe Wilhite would be a very important physician in the ER. Later and carrying us into the 2000's, would be Dr. William Beasley and his group of physicians.

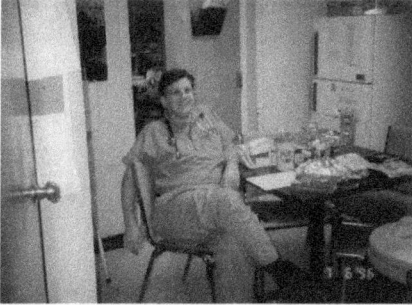

Dr. John VanDerwood

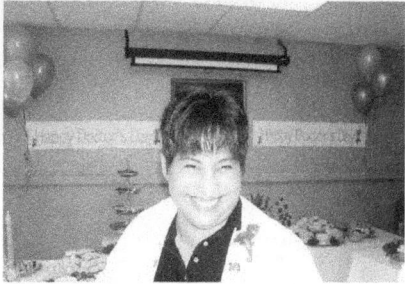

Dr. Karen Jimenez

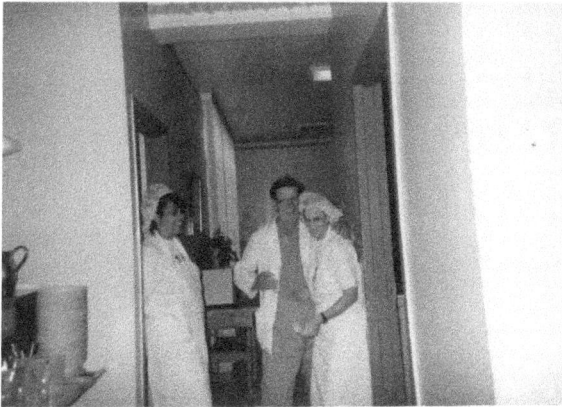

L-R: Vivian Scott, Dr. Wilhite, Donna Dearman

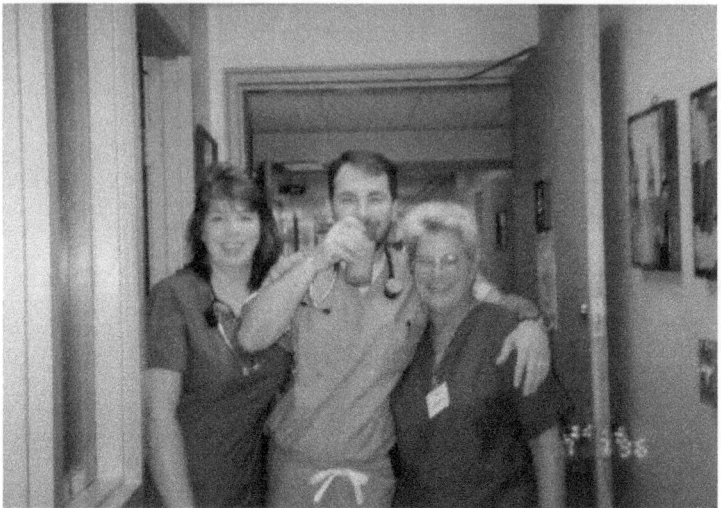

L-R: Regina Levins, Dr. Huber, Claudia Havard

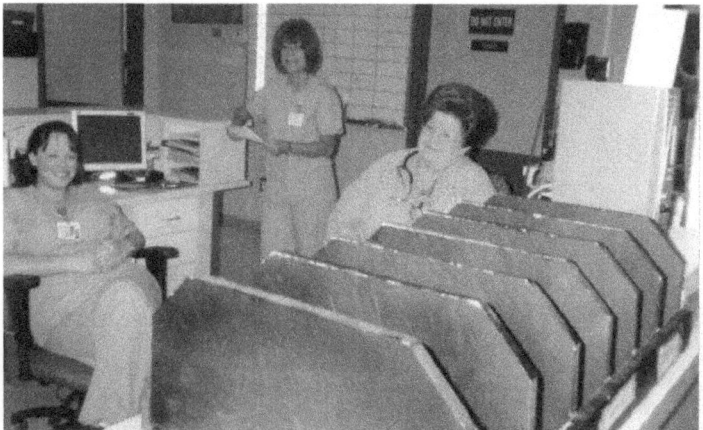

L-R: Haley Massey, Judy Mills, Paulette Dalrymple

Intensive Care

By Kathryn Cooley

In the mid-seventies, intensive care units were on the rise. George County Hospital did not have a dedicated unit. Patients who needed intensive care were monitored by a nurse who was educated for 120 hours at Mobile Infirmary. The nurse would have the patient in a room by themselves and monitor the patient on a monitor at their bedside.

The monitor was atop a crash cart which would be used if the patient's condition warranted intervention. When the decision was made to add additional space to the hospital, a four-bed intensive care unit would be built in addition to a surgical suite, obstetrics unit, central sterile unit, and recovery room.

In anticipation of the expansion, LPNs and RNs were educated and trained for the intensive care unit at Mobile Infirmary. Education included the use of all equipment, interventions, emergency drugs, use of the pacemaker, and the setup of the crash cart. All four rooms were set up the same way to reduce any potential delays in care.

A few years later, education continued to expand which included gaining certifications in advance cardiac life support (ACLS) and pediatric advanced life support (PALS).

Christine Davis and I were sent to Jackson, MS to take the ACLS course. We were two of the nurses in the class, but the majority of the class was physicians and medical students. It was a challenge, but we survived it.

The condition of some patients required additional care. The patient was usually transferred to a cardiologist in Mobile.

A transfer would require a registered nurse to handle the patient's care during transfer on the ambulance. Nursing would provide the nurses. I was the ICU supervisor; so many times I would go with the patient.

We had one patient who was needing to be transferred to Houston, TX. When I left work the day before, the patient was being transferred by ambulance. The next day, I learned he was being transferred by air. I had never flown before and that was another challenge, but we again survived.

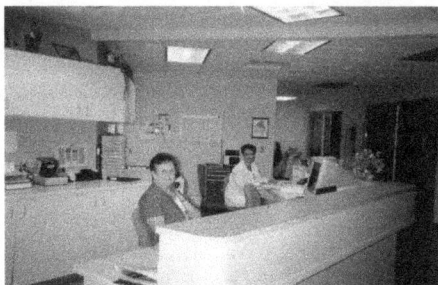

L-R: Dannie Eubanks, Gloria Havard

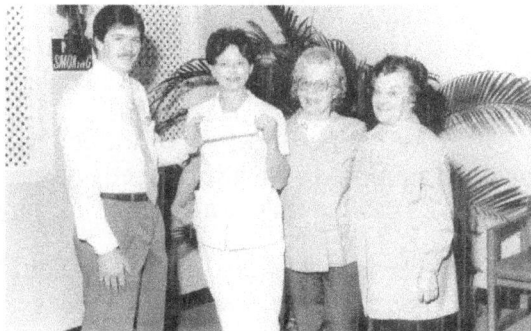

L-R: Hank Cochran, Charlotte Parnell, Lydia Havard, Volunteer

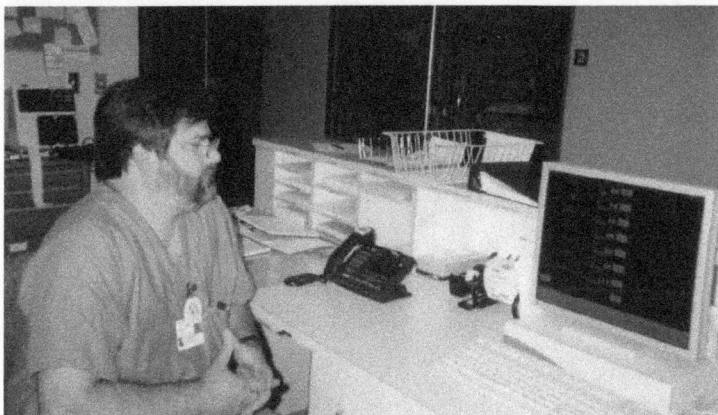

Paul May

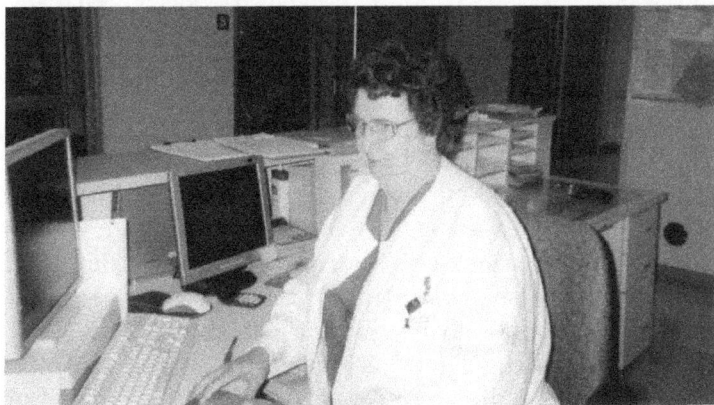

Bessie Howell

Pharmacy Services

By Carman Walley Cochran

In researching the first fifty years of the hospital pharmacy, nursing was at the forefront in the early days. I couldn't find out who was the first one in charge. But Mrs. Ruth Stonecypher is the name always associated with the pharmacy thru many of the first fifty years. She had several assistants. But the ones with longevity were Mrs. Annie Bell Strahan and Christine Stevens. Mrs. Annie Bell who was an LPN also obtained registration as a pharmacy technician with the Mississippi State Board of Pharmacy in the early nineties and came back to work in the pharmacy with the pharmacists where she was a great asset combining pharmacy with nursing care.

When the hospital first opened, a pharmacist would come by a couple times a week to verify that the medications needed were in stock and narcotics were accounted for. The first pharmacist was Mr. Larry Wozencraft. He came on staff in 1967. Mr. Larry, being the husband of the DON and having a drug store just across the street, Hospital Pharmacy, responded many times to calls during the night for needed pharmacy services. Mr. Larry is still practicing pharmacy at Beaumont Drugs in Beaumont, MS.

Mr. Al Eubanks was the second pharmacist. He also owned a drug store in town, Al's Pharmacy. Pharmacy State Board regulations were becoming more stringent. Pharmacy services still were part-time but were beginning to be needed on a more daily basis.

The medications were in the "drug room". It was kept locked, but a lot of people had the key. Shelves were on the walls all the way around the room where large stock bottles of medications were kept. This was before unit dosing. In the middle of the room was a table where the medications were prepared for dispensing to the patients. Mrs. Stonecypher would have the medications put in soufflé cups in a tray that had a notch in it to hold a 1x1 card where the name of the medication and the directions were recorded. The pharmacist would come by and verify medication accuracy and the narcotic count. The narcotics were kept in a combination safe.

Mrs. Stonecypher was very particular and wanted to make sure all State Board regulations were followed. Thirty one people had access to the pharmacy and drug cost were higher than they should have been. During the hospital renovation in the seventies the hospital bought what was called the "Brewer Machine". It was a large cabinet made by Parke Davis that would dispense medications in single doses to the nurses. It could only be accessed with a key held by the nurse and a patient card so there was a record of all doses dispensed. At the end of the first year of using the "Brewer Machine" the hospital's drug cost was reduced by fifty percent. The narcotics were moved to the nurses station in a locked box and the inventory recorded on card. Each dose dispensed would be recorded on the card with a carbon copy sheet torn off and sent to the pharmacy. The inventory was verified by nursing staff at the end of every shift.

Through the years, part-time pharmacy services were continued using the same process with many local pharmacists taking their turns keeping pharmacy services going in the hospital and in compliance with State Board of Pharmacy regulations. They performed these duties in addition to running their drugs stores or their obligations of being on staff at retail pharmacies in the area.

John T. Dressler "Butch" came on staff in 1982. He owned a local drug store, Main Drug. Melvin Fiveash came on staff in 1985. He lived locally but was the pharmacist in charge of the Walmart in Pascagoula, MS. Michael Nyman came on staff in 1988. He was the pharmacist in charge at our local Walmart and was previously on staff at Hospital Pharmacy which was a local pharmacy across the street from the hospital owned by Larry Wozencraft, Joe Taylor and Jim Dorsett. The store was originally owned by Pete Dorsett. In 1990 Rocky McGarity came on staff. He was a local pharmacist on staff at Edward's Discount Drug, owned by Mr. Hank Edwards. Rocky has since bought the store from Hank and has expanded that business.

In 1991, after the lease of the hospital ended with Mobile Infirmary, the pharmacy was contracted to Owen Healthcare, a pharmacy group located in Houston, Texas. This was the first year George County Hospital had full-time pharmacy services. Clinical services to aid the physicians were also implemented which included a hospital formulary, dosage adjustments for compromised patients, unit dosing, pharmacoeconomics, antibiogram, pharmacokinetic services, empiric therapy recommendations, policy and procedure, cart fill, floor stock, standardized administration times, laminar flow hood for sterile IV admixing, seven-day-a-week coverage and on-call services. The pharmacists in charge with Owen Healthcare were: Devon Lewis Jr. 1991, Clay Lassiter, 1991, Gino Agnelly 1992. Carman Walley Cochran was also a part-time pharmacist on staff with Owen Healthcare and on staff full time with Singing River Hospital.

When Mr. Gardner was promoted to CEO of the hospital, he started bringing in house all the ancillary services that had previously been contracted. The pharmacy department was brought under hospital management in September of 1994. Carman Walley Cochran was brought on staff as the Pharmacist in Charge and was the first full time pharmacist employed by George County Hospital.

She is still on staff today.

The pharmacy was very fortunate to have had very good technicians. Those that were on staff with the hospital pharmacy from 1994 through 2000 are: Lisa Holder, Joann Clough, Lessia Anderson, Annie Bell Strahan, Donnis Byrd, Dustin Walley and Joshua Jordan.

As the hospital continued to expand services, the pharmacy department was moved in the latter nineties to the Joyce Cochran Chapel because space was very limited. The "drug room" was converted to the "Scope Room" where colonoscopies were performed.

Through the years, the hospital has worked closely and as partners with the local pharmacies listed above and also with one not mentioned, Jim's Discount Drug owned and operated by Jim Busby and his son Pat. The Busbys have always been an asset to the hospital.

We would like to thank all the pharmacists, technicians and pharmacies in our town for assisting the hospital in providing patient care for the patients of George County Hospital.

We would also like to thank Dr. Whites for always being there to lead and guide and support all the pharmacies' efforts to provide good patient care.

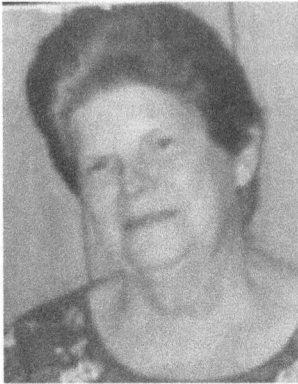

Anabelle Strahan

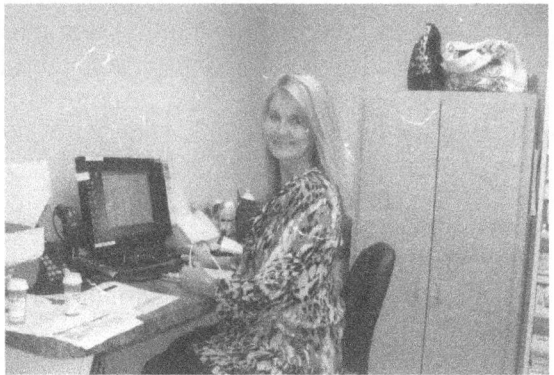

Carman Walley Cochran

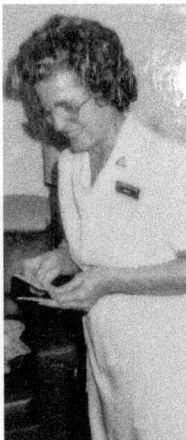

Ruth Stonecypher

Ambulance Service

By Dr. Dayton Whites and Christine Davis

When George County Hospital opened in 1950, there was no ambulance service available in the George County area. In 1956, George County funeral home purchased a DeSoto station wagon which had been converted into a small ambulance.

There was no one, at that time, who waited by the phone to dispatch an ambulance to an emergency. When accidents occurred, the Sheriff's Department usually summoned the ambulance. The ambulance was used to transfer patients from home or from accident sites to the emergency room. Also, the same vehicle was used to transfer sick patients from George County Hospital to one of the larger hospitals in our area.

In 1966, Sheriff Eugene Howell established an ambulance service for George County. During this period of time, a person could get ambulance service by calling the number listed in the phone directory. This service did not work very well because it only offered a driver. Help was on a volunteer basis and those volunteering knew very little about taking care of sick or injured patients.

In the early 70's, George County Hospital assumed the responsibility of ambulance services for George County and its area. They purchased two van-type ambulances. The van ambulances were stocked with medical supplies and contained one stretcher. A portable stretcher could be situated parallel on the other side in the event of multiple patient injuries. The patient was strapped in, but the employees did not wear seat belts during that time. After a period of time, the hospital purchased a modular type ambulance with more modern equipment and the capability to provide care for critically ill or injured patients.

Hospital employees were responsible for manning the ambulance. A driver, a nurse or other medically trained personnel, were the crew. If heavy lifting was involved, the male attendant on duty for the hospital would also go.

Christine was very involved in managing the hospital's busy ambulance service and became George County's first female ambulance driver. She also worked as an emergency room nurse, obstetrical nurse and floor nurse during that period. Most of the drivers actually worked in other departments of the hospital and some worked in law enforcement. No special license was required to drive ambulances.

The nurses were pulled from the emergency room or the floor if an ambulance was needed. If their uniform got soaked or soiled, they were given surgical scrubs to wear for the remainder of their shift. There were no paramedics at that time but many hospital employees took an EMT (Emergency Medical Technician) course that was taught locally by a young man named Tim Bailey. Mr. Bailey was responsible for implementing the first EMT program to be taught in George County.

The ambulances were very busy. The calls included nursing home and hospital transfers, at-home pickups for illness or injury and, of course, motor vehicle accidents. There were many wrecks on a one major highway that traversed our county which garnered it the name "Bloody 98".

During football season, the ambulance and crew were at all home games and were often utilized to provide emergency treatment or transport of injured football players. The community embraced this service provided by the hospital. The services continued to grow and improve the medical care provided to George County citizens.

In 1981, Mike Henderson was hired to be in charge of the ambulance department for George County Hospital. With his leadership, the qualifications changed. The driver was required to have a commercial license and if possible, some medical background. The medical person accompanying the driver was required to have an ACLS certification.

In 1985, Mobile Infirmary took over the management for the hospital which included the ambulance service. Mr. Henderson continued to oversee the ambulance services during this time.

In 1989, George County again assumed the responsibility of ownership and management of George County Hospital and the ambulance services. Mr. Henderson continued to be in charge until 1992. Few major changes were made in the service until 1996.

In 1996, after retiring from the military, Park Tritle was hired to run the ambulance service and did so for the next 10 years.

During the first 50 years of operation the people with George County Hospital emergency services made great strides in the provision of medical care and transport of the critically ill or injured in the county and surrounding areas. The ambulance service proved to be a vital component and valuable asset of George County Hospital.

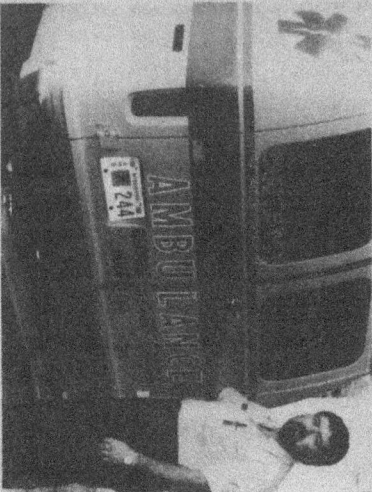

THURSDAY, DECEMBER 18, 1986

GEORGE COUNTY TIMES, LUCEDALE, MISSISSIPPI 39452

PAGE FIFTEEN

On 24-Hour Standby... GEORGE COUNTY HOSPITAL Ambulance Supervisor Mike Henderson explains that the ambulance service is on standby 24 hours a day, seven days a week.

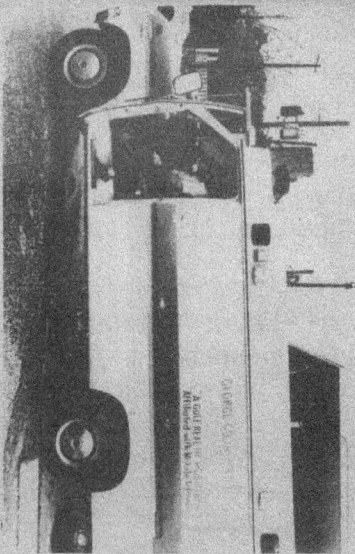

Ambulance... MIKE HENDERSON, driver and supervisor of the George County Hospital ambulance service, states that both of the hospital's ambulances can carry up to four patients on each trip to the hospital.

(Photos by Joy M. Hart)

Dietary Department

By Susan Turner and Patsy Smith

When the hospital opened in 1950, the kitchen and dining room were located in the same space they are in today. Not much changed in the first fifty years. Mrs. Barr was the dietician for years. Employees served themselves from pots of food placed on the table by the stove in the kitchen. Meals were free.

In 1967, a steam table was installed, allowing dietary workers to serve the food. At this time, meal tickets were purchased for five dollars each. Different amounts were written around the edges of the tickets. Prices started at five cents and went up to forty cents. If you ate lightly, tickets would last for several days.

The food was cooked from scratch by wonderful cooks. Some of the cooks were Bessie Morse, Vera Mae McDowell, and Margaret Havard. Other workers were Choicie Miles, Birdia Mae Grant, Mae Ruth Hill, Georgia Mae Ludgood, and Lillie Maude Williams. On fried-chicken days, people would gladly wait in a long line to get a piece of their delicious fried chicken. Bessie Morse was famous for her chicken and dumplings and bread pudding. The food was always wonderful.

Amy Boutwell, registered dietician, came to work in 1965. Doris Dickson Pope was hired as a dietary assistant. Mrs. Pope was able to take a course to become a certified dietary assistant. Mrs. Boutwell retired in 1969. Susan Turner, a registered dietician, took over but eventually resigned in

1977.

At that time, Carolyn Bailey worked for several years. Then, Lanell Kirkpatrick, registered dietician, was contracted as a private dietary consultant. Doris Pope retired in 1986. Then Vera Havard, a dietary assistant, worked until she retired. She was replaced by Keith Stinson.

Breakfast was served each morning at 7:30. Late trays were served for N.P.O. patients or new admissions. Lunch was at 11:30 and supper was at 5:30. Juice, crackers, or cookies were offered at night for patients. Food was always left out for the 11-7 shifts. Different menus had to be planned for approximately eleven different types of diets.

The dining room had five tables that seated four people to each table and a large conference table for hospital trustees, who met there for their monthly meetings.

George County Hospital was blessed with great dietary workers, great cooks, and great food. The first shift was 6:00 a.m. to 2:00 p.m. and the second shift was from 10:30 a.m. to 6:30 p.m.

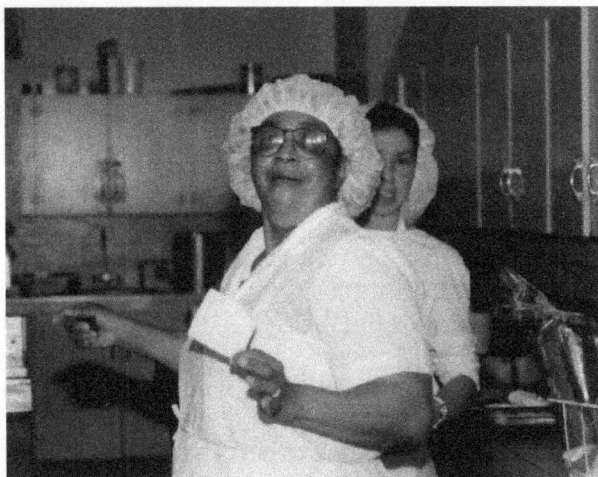

Mae Ruth Hill

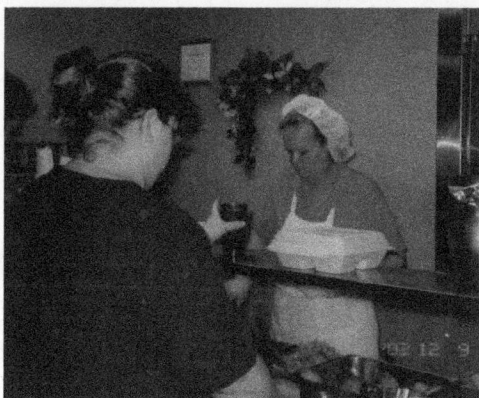

Ella Erkhart

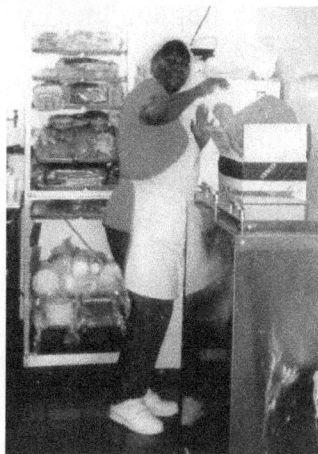

Georgia Dorsey

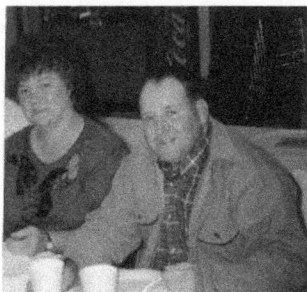

Susan Turner (husband Phil)

Business Office

By Patsy Smith

February of 1961 was the beginning of my lifelong career at George County Hospital. I was a nurse aide. Little did I know, I would not retire until 39 years later in May of 2000. When I first began working, Hazel Croom was the administrator and Inez Harmon was the director of nurses. At that time, when a patient needed assistance, they turned on their call light which then turned on a light over their door. We then had to walk to the room to see what was needed, retrieve whatever it was, and return to the room. There were no bathrooms in the first semi-private rooms. This made bed pans a necessity.

The duties for a nurse aide consisted of bed baths, linen changing, administering therapeutic treatments, and taking vital signs for patients who came into the emergency room. If you worked the 3-11 or 11-7 shifts, you would also have to prep the OBs for delivery and clean the delivery rooms. There was one labor room and one delivery room. Nurse aides also attended to newborn babies in the nursery, which was located next to Nurse Desk #1. There was no assigned nursery nurse and everyone worked wherever they were needed. One of the benefits at this time was that workers could eat free. The 11-7 shift could use the kitchen to cook. This gave me the opportunity to learn how to fry chicken with the help of Mrs. Ruby Bishop, RN.

The purchasing department consisted of one room across from the kitchen. Corrine Morgan, LPN did the purchasing and dispersing of medical and surgical supplies. As the hospital grew, purchasing was moved to a new building behind the hospital which also housed the maintenance department and a laundry.

Earl Hudson was the maintenance man. He also retrieved the mail from the post office each day. Earl was a dedicated employee for many years and was always willing to do anything needed.

In 1964, I was transferred to the business office by Keith Scott, the administrator at that time. The business office consisted of two separate offices. It was located at the front of the hospital next to the front lobby. The administrator's office was just across the hall. There were five workers in the business office: Willene Johnson, insurance clerk, Vera Havard, admissions clerk, Dorothea Hunter, bookkeeper, Helen Cowart and Ella Stevens, medical records. I made the sixth employee as another admissions clerk. I was also trained by Dorothea Hunter to help with payroll and accounts payable. Horace Bradley, CPA, was hospital auditor. I was soon transferred to Dorothea Hunter's position upon her becoming ill and resigning. All patient accounting, accounts payable, and payroll had to be done by hand in large ledger books.

Medicare and Medicaid were signed into law in July of 1965. Medicare covered senior citizens. Medicaid covered low-income families, pregnant women, people of all ages with disabilities, and people in need of long-term care. These health programs brought about change to the way we filed insurance. This required more personnel. The new hires were: Helen Croom, Vernon Goff, Pat Horne, Geraldine Williams, Carrie Wells, Mary Helen McKinnley, and Marci Cumberland. Many changes had to be made in insurance and patient billing also. Horace Bradley, Willene Johnson and I went to Jackson to learn guidelines for filing insurance claims.

Other advancements were also added to the hospital such as a switchboard to connect calls to patient rooms.

High school students were hired to work part-time on the switchboard. Mary Lou Tipton was our first medical transcriptionist. Doctors' discharge notes and patient histories were hand written before this time.

In 1976, we received our first Burroughs bookkeeping machine. Patient charges, accounts payable, and payroll were stored in a strip on a card. This made it quicker and easier to keep our records. It was about this time that a new outpatient office was opened with a much smaller switchboard. This new office was open 24/7. One of the first outpatient clerks was Dessie Leggett. Dessie was confined to a wheelchair due to an automobile accident. But she was still dedicated to her job. Other switchboard employees were Mae Jewel Dixon, Julia Havard, and Hannalore Parker.

A new emergency room was soon added, allowing extra space for incoming patients. We also had an ER nurse for all three shifts. In the early 1980s, we were having a cash-flow problem. Some office employees were cut back to four days a week. It was a day-to-day struggle to keep the bills paid. Payroll and payroll taxes always had to be paid. There was one administrator who decided he needed his wife to take on my job as office manager and accounts payable. I was moved to the purchasing department to replace someone who had been doing a good job.

After several months, the hospital was placed on C.O.D. We had to have a check ready when a delivery was made and I had to go to Mobile with a check to pick up supplies. This administrator was gone and the person he had put in my position picked up her purse and left, leaving no one to do her job. There were unpaid bills and unopened mail going back for months. Everything was a mess. I was taken into the administrator's office by two hospital board members and asked if I would try to get the office back in order. They said they couldn't promise me a permanent position, but I accepted the offer regardless.

There had been a new accounting system installed and I had to wait for someone to come from Jackson to train me. They had no idea how badly we were in debt. It took me at least two weeks to be trained and to get all of the mail opened and entered into the system. When a cost-requirements list was run, the hospital owed over $400,000. I was never moved back to Purchasing. I remained in the business office as its office manager doing accounts payable and whatever else had to be done.

I have many fond memories of my tenure at the hospital. For two years, we had a choir of hospital workers who sang Christmas carols on the front steps of the hospital. Dr. Tipton was a member of the choir.

I loved the hospital. I loved my job and always counted it a privilege to have been a part of George County Hospital. During my 39 years, I witnessed many changes, worked under fifteen different administrators, and made lasting friends who became like family. I will always cherish my time as an employee of George County Hospital.

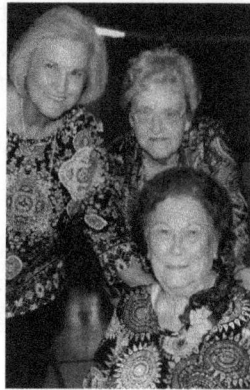

Back row: Pat Horne and Patsy Smith
Front: Helen Ruth Croom

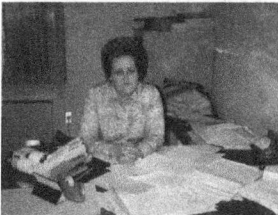

Patsy Smith

Medical Record Department

By Christy Edwards Roberts, RHIA, CHPS, CHC

The medical record department kicked off in royal style as the hospital opened. Ample space was given to the department to set up clerical desks, typewriter stations, shelving units, manual log books, cabinets for index card storage and other filing paperwork. The department received premium space at the very front of the facility. It is believed that the department may be the only area which hasn't moved in the first 50 years of business!

Our first medical record custodian was Helen Cowart. Over the first fifty years, we've only had a total of seven people in this leadership role: Helen Cowart, Ella Stevens, Margaret Williams, Gean Davis, Christy Edwards Roberts, RHIA, Lynn Sheldon and Shanon Roberts. The art of medical record science is a fun and challenging career path. To be successful in this role requires someone to be organized, good with numbers/statistics, can follow the rules set forth by the regulatory agencies (both state and federal), read legible and illegible written documentation alike, good sense of humor, patience (or the ability to cultivate it), multitasking extraordinaire, a good communicator and knowing a doctors favorite food is a plus. Food is an age-old strategy to get physicians to complete their charts (haha).

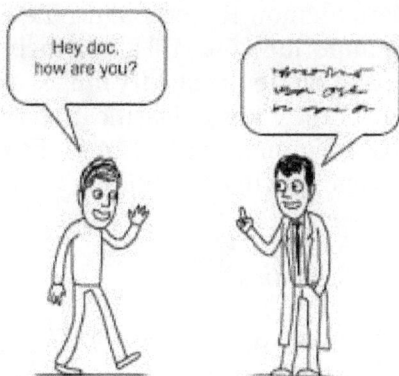

A Day in the Life

A routine day in the 1950's consisted of the following: lots of paper, pens/pencils, index cards and walking around the hospital delivering or picking up mail, bills to drop, dictation, 1,000 interruptions, phone to answer (maybe even the switchboard depending on your hospital), admissions to register, discharges to depart, census of patients to type up and deliver, questions to answer for visitors and staff, meetings, take old records to the floor for physician review, complete birth and death certificates, evaluate documents for deficiencies, etc. A list of new, current and discharged patients had to be documented daily for inpatients, outpatients, surgery and emergency room. The breaking point used to tally this data was and still is midnight.

Coding & DRGs

During the early years of the department, one person generally performed all of the duties. It wasn't until the early 1980's that the department really started to grow. In 1983 the government started a new payment strategy for inpatients call diagnosis related groups (DRGs). This required additional personnel to accomplish the task. Paulette Dairy and Donna Pate were the first two individuals to hold the DRG/coder title in the department and others during these years were Shanon Roberts and Linda Holland. DRGs were very important and still are in their form today. The inpatient payment to the facility hinges on this individual's knowledge of the coding classification system and the resulting DRG assignment based upon the codes they select from the physician's documentation within the record.

Statistics

The first baby born at the hospital was on 9/6/1950. It was a boy! Dr. R. L. Benson delivered the baby, and the parents gave their child the middle name of Benson. We presume to honor the delivering physician. We have always been required to keep and submit birth and death information to the state vital records division. We also are required to report certain communicable diseases to the state. Oncology (cancer) reporting wasn't required until 1996.

General hospital statistics are still a foundation task within the department: census, patient days, volume by department or area, insurance or financial class, doctor, procedures, etc. We track this information and can give totals by the day, month, quarter, calendar or fiscal year according to what the requestor needs. This type of information combined with payment data is used for profit/ loss analysis just as it would in any other line of business.

Dictation and Transcription

It all began with someone somewhere having poor handwriting. In a quest to read a physician's handwriting after the ink had dried, a transcriptionist was born. Then the physician just had to talk and the transcriptionist legibly wrote it down.

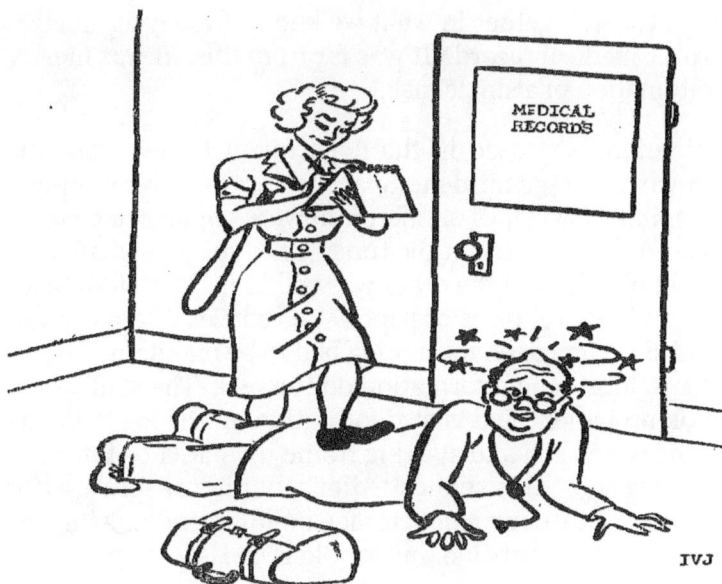

HOW TO TRAP DOCTORS FOR DICTATION

Our facility made its first major dictation advancement in 1988. We purchased an endless loop dictation tape system. The physicians really embraced the technology because it made their work more efficient. They could just pick up a dedicated phone and dictate what they needed the transcriptionists to type and be on their way.

The first transcriptionist hired for the department was Mary Lou Tipton. Over the years these ladies also typed for us: Sharon Snellgrove, Pam Davis, Jean Parnell, Janice Grant, Barbara Holland, Wynette Hare, Rose Heathcoe, Sherry Williams, Sherry Eubanks, Gean Davis and Shelia Bataglia.

Computerization

Over the first 50 years the hospital, and department, would primarily be paper based and very scant technology was in place. That doesn't mean that each department didn't have some technology, because it did, but it wasn't all meshed together in what we know of today as an electronic medical record. It was far from this. It was merely automation of a single task.

Microfilm was used in the department to help ease the growing storage burden. Space is always a premium in a hospital! Two types of microfilm were popular in medical record departments at the time. One type was small 4 x 5 sheet of fiche and the other was roll film. Microfilm takes a standard size piece of paper and reduces it to a thumbnail sized image. A master log had to be maintained in order to locate the information on the reel. The staff would look up patient and visit information on the log to determine which roll and starting frame the patient's information was on. This sounds tedious, but it was far superior to digging through a hot storage building and moving box after box for hours looking for old records.

In 1990 the hospital received a proposal from Data Systems Management for computerization in the admission, medical record, business office, inventory, payroll and general ledger. The system was designed to run using an IBM 36 computer and the AS400 server. A memo was located from the company regarding the integration of faxing to the system starting January 1, 1994. The IBM system was not replaced until 2003.

Release of Information

Physicians and patients alike have always been able to request copies of medical records. Confidentiality of medical information has always been of high importance to anyone in the healthcare community. But, as a testament to the close-knit community and lack of early privacy laws, each morning patient names were read aloud on our local radio station, WRBE. Everyone in the county listened to the radio station to see who was in the hospital each day. The sharing of this information would lead to many visits from friends and family members and lots of cooking for the family members of sick patients.

Closing

The Medical Record staff members wear many hats, so to speak. Over the years we have enjoyed the diversity of the department and the growing pains associated with our first fifty years. The comradery with the other staff members and physicians has made all the twists and turns worth the while.

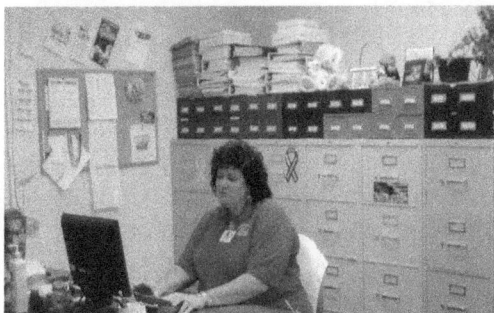

Marci Cumberland

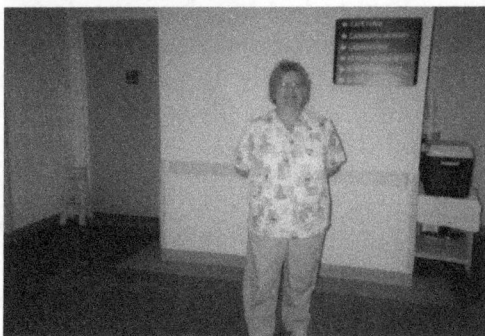

Janice Grant

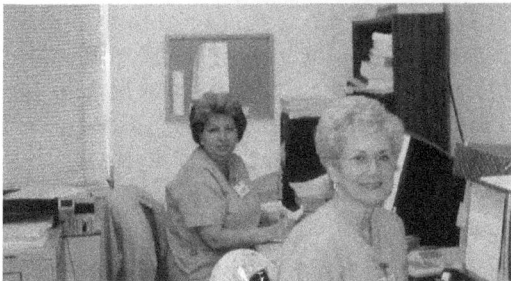

Shanon Roberts and Gean Davis

Is It A Joke?

by Shanon Roberts

Once when transcribing dictation for Dr. Shaw, I had Pam Davis one of our transcriptionist ask me to come and listen to the recording. Dr. Shaw was instructing us to send a copy of the report to a physician in Jackson. Dr. Shaw called him Dr. Condom. He sounded serious, but we thought surely he is playing a joke. Dr. Shaw did have a keen sense of humor. We had to ask to be certain. The physician's lounge is located next to medical records, so I told Pam to just knock on the door and ask. I can still hear all the physicians laughing at us. They thought our concern and chagrin about the name was hilarious. Thing is, the Dr.'s name really was Condom.

UNFAMILIAR ACCENT!

On one occasion we had a new OB/GYN, Dr. Kornstein join the staff. He had a heavy accent. There is always a learning curve when you start transcribing for a new doctor, but his accent made it a little more difficult for us. On his first operative report, I had Janice Grant just type what she thought it sounded like. We were not able to understand several phrases. I took the report to his office and waited to speak with him in person. I wanted him to educate us on the procedure and his phrasing. I told him I know you did not say "throw the uterus in the trash," but what did you say? To my embarrassment he leaned back in his chair to laugh then leaned forward on his desk to laugh, no, no it was "the uterus was retracted." Thankfully he just thought it was very, very funny. He was gracious in working with us until we mastered his accent.

HIPAA

With HIPAA the rules for release of information changed greatly. No longer could we just honor a subpoena, we had to notify all parties involved. This gives all parties an opportunity to have their attorney quash the subpoena until further directions by a judge. The only subpoena we could honor without notifying all parties was by court order signed by a judge. It is sad to say that medical record personnel was educated on this law before legal personnel was. The first group of subpoenas we received after this new regulation came without being by court order, therefore I notified all parties involved. Within several days I had an irate judge call me for doing this. Several of the subpoenas were for criminal cases even though they were not by court order. He threatened me with obstruction of justice, seems I had caused" all the criminals to run away." He was so upset. When I tried to explain this regulation he threatened to prosecute me, unless I could prove this new law to him. THANK GOODNESS FOR THE FEDERAL REGISTER AND OUR CONSULTANT. I can find humor in this now and hopefully the judge can too, but I have to say that it was stressful situation until the legal system caught up with government regulations on HIPAA.

ONE ON MYSELF

Long before I began working in medical records, I was part of nursing service. I started my career as a student in the Health Occupation Program that was part of the George County High School in 1975. Seniors were allowed to work partial days at the hospital as part of this program. I loved it. I was assigned to work in the ER. All went well for several days, then we had a patient who came in with a very large, gaping wound of the scalp. I helped clean and shave the wound for suturing, no problem. Then Dr. Tipton placed me behind him to watch the suturing process. Did you know, in a wound such as this, when you inject

Lidocaine into the scalp, the needle will lift the flap up and away from the bone? First injection, fine, second injection fine, I don't know about the third injection, it was at that time I decided to check out. The next thing I remember was a flurry of people helping me up and placing me on a stool. Dr. Tipton was still injecting the scalp, but he told everyone to calm down saying she did exactly what I instructed her to do. I told her to "lay on the floor and play ghost." Don't judge me too harshly, I was only seventeen! I went on to work as a nurse for many years, and saw much worse than the scalp wound without ever fainting again.

Physical Therapy

By Johnny Smith

I began working in Lucedale in June 1991 as a contract therapist with Sunbelt Therapy. GCH at that time had been contracting physical therapy with Sunbelt. A typical day would be a combination of wound care, three or four outpatients, and some acute-care inpatients.

My hospital day was usually done by 2:00 p.m. I would do home health with South Mississippi Home Health the rest of the day. On occasion, I would need to come back to the hospital to do another patient, but that was rare.

Once a week, I would make early morning rounds with the doctors, usually Dr. Whites and/or Dr. Shaw. This was fascinating to me. I got a chance to see how they thought and interacted with their patients. I enjoyed this very much.

The outpatient care was rather similar to anywhere else with the exception of the wound care. I got to see and work with a wide variety of patients that I would not have seen in most other facilities. The surgeon, Dr. Suresh, was excellent at referring patients to therapy, including burn victims. I loved this.

Around June 1994, the contract with Sunbelt was not re-newed by the hospital. So, Sunbelt opened their clinic on Mill Street. I worked there until November 1996. During this time, Paul Gardner, CEO of the Hospital, indicated to me that he wanted to open a therapy and wellness center. Eventually, I agreed to come to work as a hospital employee and to open what became Southeast Rehab and Wellness Center on Mill Street in Lucedale.

On January 6, 1997, I became an employee of the George County Hospital system. Initially, we were in the same place at the hospital as when I contracted. During 1997, we had a team that was looking into wellness center equipment and, of course, I worked on ordering the equipment for Southeast Rehab.

Around December 1, 1997, the therapy department opened at Southeast Rehab. As far as I can remember, we began offering occupational and speech therapy too. However, wound care and inpatient care remained at the hospital for the next few years.

At some point, we expanded into Greene County with all three therapies. But I'm not sure if it was before 2000.

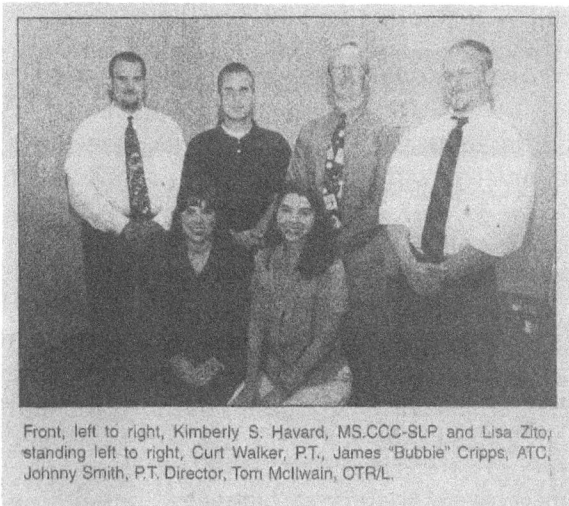

Front, left to right, Kimberly S. Havard, MS.CCC-SLP and Lisa Zito; standing left to right, Curt Walker, P.T., James "Bubbie" Cripps, ATC, Johnny Smith, P.T. Director, Tom McIlwain, OTR/L.

Cardiopulmonary/Respiratory

By Lendon Elmore

I came to work at the hospital in 1989. I was hired by Joe McNulty, the owner of Medicomp, a provider of Respiratory Services and equipment. George County Hospital was financially challenged at that time and the administration figured the best way for them to offer qualify respiratory services, was to contract out these services, though Medicomp.

On my first day of work, J.P. Byrd, the previous director, had already taken a job elsewhere and things were kind of in limbo. Kathy Stegall, a wonderful employee, was doing a great job of holding down the fort. Two OJTs, Lance and Frank, rounded out the crew. The department was in one small room with two desks, an ABG machine, supplies, and a coffee pot. We hardly had room to turn around in, but we made it work. There was plenty to do, so we hit the ground running.

From the beginning, we offered a full range of respiratory services and equipment. But, due to financial constraints, the respiratory department's in-house hours were limited to day shift 0700-1900, Monday through Friday. Call was taken for after hours.

After hours, the nurses were great about doing routine aerosol treatments, O2 setups, and an occasional EKG. But when it was an emergency or something outside of their expertise, the nurse would initiate a call-back to the respiratory therapist on call.

The unpredictable nature of call-backs was quite a challenge. We were responsible and prepared to be called back in for "bad" COPD patients, ventilator rounds, ventilator alarms and code 100s, just to name a few. At that time, I lived within a couple blocks of the hospital, so that helped a lot. We were very busy and worked with a limited staff. Many times, after working some of the night, we would be there for the following day shift.

Respiratory call-ins were unacceptable, unless YOU were a patient in the hospital. Respiratory staff car trouble? No problem. I would come pick you up.

Back then, doctors Whites, Shaw and the rest of the doctors took their turns working in the Emergency Department and responding to codes. If a situation arose that would require a patient to be intubated, and no nurse anesthetist was available, respiratory therapists would directly assist the doctor, and on many occasions, when asked, would intubate the patients.

The attitude back then, seemingly shared by all the employees, was, if there was an immediate need, you would jump in and help, even if outside your immediate responsibilities.

At that time, George County Hospital had its own ambulance service. Many people, from all disciplines, became ambulance drivers. They made it work. There were times, when a critical patient was having trouble breathing and needed transfer by ambulance, a respiratory therapist and a nurse would accompany them, bagging the patient along the way.

In those early days, the shaky financial situation played on the background. There were a couple of times the liquid O2 tanks that supplied the hospital were not filled and we had to go to the backup cylinders.

There were, and still are, a lot of dedicated, caring employees choosing this hospital as their workplace. Back then, some maybe took it a little more personally. A couple of examples come to mind. Bessie Howell: We knew she would be calling us if we were five minutes late for an aerosol treatment, always wanting to know if we were on our way. Dr. Suresh could be very intense. He called me once about a late incentive spirometer on one of his patients. (We were in a code.) I assured him we would be there ASAP. He said just let him know if we could not make it, because he would do it himself.

We became official employees of George County Hospital on October 27, 1993, when administrator Paul Gardner, bought us out of the contract with Medicomp. Finances were better at the hospital, and we expanded our hours to 24/7 and were able to purchase much-needed equipment.

A short while later, we moved Echo and Vascular Ultrasound under our umbrella and renamed the department 'Cardiopulmonary'.

About two years ago, we opened George Regional Sleep Services. We've been very successful in helping many people with their sleep-associated problems.

We have a great group of employees providing service in the Cardiopulmonary Department. I know it's true because employees from other departments stop me and tell me that all the time.

Karen Saussy is the assistant director. The Cardiopulmonary department consists of her, Susan Read, Deanna Reynolds, Tammy Ehlers, Paige Dykes, Marvin North, and several key PRN employees. The Echo and Vascular Department has Darlene Emerson as its supervisor and Alexis Styron as staff. The Sleep Services Lab employs Cris Lambert who does a wonderful job.

I consider myself lucky to have played a small role in the chapter of the book of works here at George County (now Regional) Hospital.

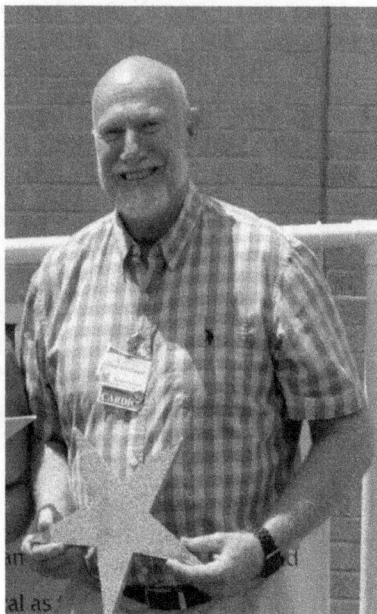

Lendon Elmore

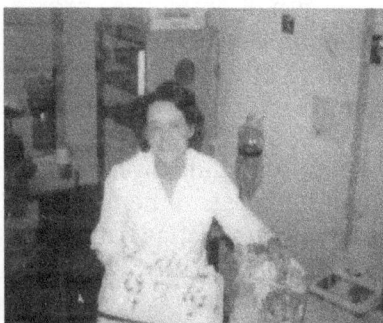

Joyce Cochran

Unit/Ward Clerks

1970-1988

By Doris Jean Eckhoff

I cannot recall the exact dates, but this is close. We had two nursing stations. Each had a ward clerk. If I am correct, we had six. There was one for each (7a-3p, 3p-11p, 11p-7a) eight-hour shift with others as relief in case someone had to have requested off days or sickness. Our titles were 'ward clerks'. Later, we were given the title 'unit secretary'.

Back in these days, our main job was first learning to read the physicians' writing. Each time one of the physicians admitted a patient, our main job was to make sure we wrote out the correct diagnosis and all of the required requests. There were several requests for different departments. All of this was done by hand. There were no such things as computers.

All of this was done and checked by the RN for accuracy. After this was completed, all of the requests were delivered by foot to each department. After the requests were completed, the requests were all returned to the proper places to be placed on the proper charts. These were to be placed on the charts in order for the physician to help confirm their diagnosis.

These things were fairly simple after you caught on. Another simple task was keeping new sheets in each chart so the physicians could write new orders. Once, we heard a calamity. As we looked up, a chart came sliding down the hall (angry physician). After that episode, we were more careful to make sure there was plenty of space for new doctor's orders. This mistake never happened again.

This was a very interesting place of employment. I was employed there almost 15 years. I learned a lot about different medications and diseases.

We had fun times and sad times. There were also trying times, especially losing people you had grown up with. My dad passed away while I was employed there.

Everyone, including the physicians, was like one big, happy family.

Those of us still living enjoy meeting up with former employees and talking about the old times at George County Hospital.

Other long-time ward clerks include: Janelle Moore, Geneva Gibson, Vondell Evans, Donnis Byrd, Debbie Stinson, Doris Rone, and Gladys Davis.

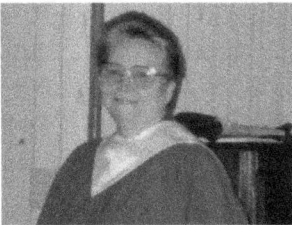

Donnis Byrd

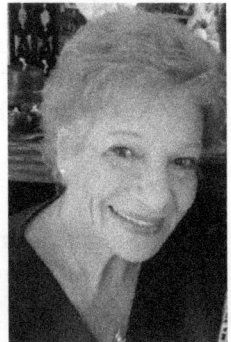

Geneva Gibson

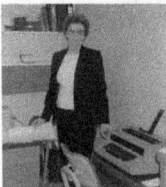

Doris Jean Eckhoff

Communication

By The Committee

When George County Hospital opened in 1950, it opened with the same phone number that it uses today, 947-3161. At first, all calls coming into the hospital were answered at a small switchboard located in the business office. Marie Weaver was the first operator on the switchboard. When the business office closed each day, all calls were answered at the nurse's desk. Besides the phone at nurse's station, there were phones located in the operating room, emergency room, laboratory, x-ray department, the business office and the administrator's office.

In 1964, George County Hospital placed phones in each patient's room. Phone system wise, things remain the same until 1977 when the emergency room waiting room and outpatient office with communication space was added. With this, all incoming calls, 24 hours a day, were answered in the outpatient office. Calls to patients in the hospital were handled through this office and in hospital phone communication was all also cared for in this new phone system.

In the late 1970s, beeper service became a part of communication for George County Hospital. This allowed a way for the hospital to be able to get in touch with doctors on staff as well as emergency personnel when needed. Through this service, a phone number appeared on the beeper. By calling that phone number, needed information was received. This service was used for more than 10 years.

George County Hospital took over the 911 system in the early 90s. This was set up in the communication room in the emergency room. This worked very well and was used until the system was moved to the George County Courthouse.

Employees who were involved in the communication system of George County Hospital for many years and did an excellent job were Dessie Leggett, Mae Jewel Dixon and Hannalore Parker.

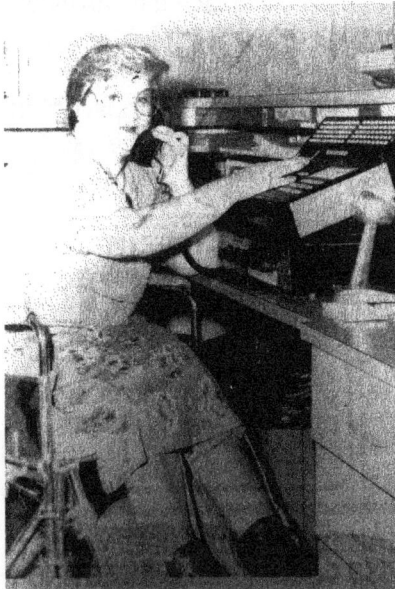

Dessie Leggett at switchboard

Maintenance

By the Committee

The early days in the George County Hospital Maintenance Department were much different than those 5 decades later. Initially, diagnosis and treatment techniques at our hospital, even much larger hospitals, were very primitive. For instance, the laboratory department performed no more than 10 to 15 different procedures. These consisted of using the microscope and performing chemical processes by hand. All X-rays were still images, as there was no such thing as fluoroscopy. Intravenous treatment was in the early stages and very few medications were given intravenously. The rate of fluid infusions was set manually by the nurse in charge and the timeframe to complete an infusion was somewhat of a guess. There were no IV pumps, no sophisticated lab or radiology equipment requiring maintenance.

Hospital maintenance essentially consisted of maintaining the electrical, water and sewer systems. The Maintenance Department was also in charge of grounds-keeping. The first full-time maintenance employee was Mr. Earl Hudson. In addition to the maintenance and odd jobs that arose, he would lend a hand in the kitchen, on the hall, or in housekeeping, where ever there was a need. He is remembered fondly as a great asset to the facility

As years passed, diagnostic and treatment modalities became more complex. Modern equipment was purchased to meet the needs of a rapidly growing community. The Laboratory and Radiological capabilities expanded, but still the Maintenance Department was not responsible for their equipment. The companies who sold the equipment trained the employees operating the equipment how to use and maintain it.

With the 1977 addition and renovation of George County Hospital, things began to change for the Maintenance Department. A growing facility, now had an ICU/CCU. A larger surgical department, modernization of the older areas and increased maintenance demands heralded the era of Mr. Benny Wall. Mr. Wall was in charge of the Maintenance Department for several years. He was extremely knowledgeable and a quick study. He was capable of learning how to take care of almost any problem that arose with the facility or the equipment. Everyone had great confidence in his abilities and he was a great mentor to his crew. Along this same time two other memorable maintenance employees were George Henderson and Bob Chisholm.

Mr. Alton Neel was hired in this position after Mr. Wall left. He continued to carry out the day to day duties of maintaining a facility with 24 hour a day, 7 days a week operation. All the moving parts, some newer and a lot getting older required repair, replacement and maintenance. Mr. Neel and crew performed these duties and kept the facility running like a finely tuned machine.

In 1993 Mr. Mike Hutchison was hired. He renovated the building where the hospital Wellness Center is located on Mill Street as well as the office of the new surgeon, Dr. Suresh. Along with his construction duties, he also directed the Maintenance Department. He and his crew were in charge of a growing facility with increasing architectural maintenance requirements as well technological systems installation and upkeep. His tenure in this department brought us up to and well past the year 2000.

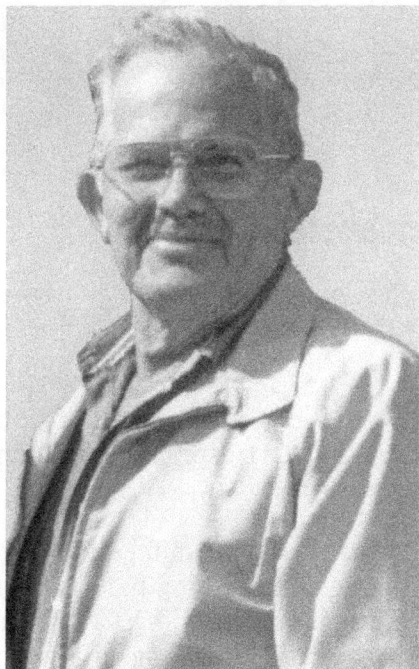

Bennie Wall

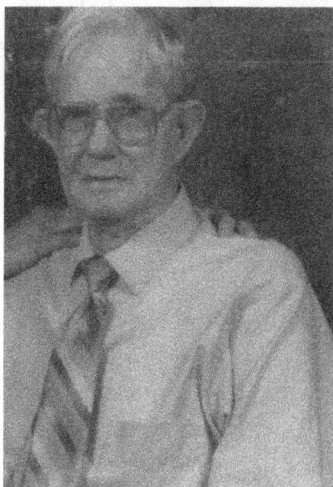

Earl Hudson

Housekeeping

By The Committee

It was very hard to get information concerning the history of housekeeping at George County Hospital. No present employees worked prior to 2001.

Early in the history of George County Hospital, the charge nurse was basically in charge of everything that went on during her shift. This included the cleanliness of all the hospital rooms and halls. At the beginning, the 7 – 3 shift changed all beds for the new day. Basically, at the time, there were two employee groups who took care of the cleanliness of the hospital. The female personnel were called nurse's aides and the male personnel were called orderlies. The nurse's aides were responsible for making beds each morning. They also took care of the cleanliness of their patients and their room. The orderlies' job was to take care of male patients. The orderly on 11 to 7 shift was responsible for keeping the halls cleaned and floors waxed.

In other words, George County Hospital did not have a housekeeping department since it was taken care of by the nursing staff. Wauldine King was hired in the late 1950's. She took a leadership role in housekeeping and made strides in organizing a housekeeping department. Following this, Lydia Havard was hired in the late 1960's to head of department. She put together plans and people to make a good independent housekeeping department.

As the hospital became larger, so did housekeeping. Through the years, this department has kept up with current cleaning techniques and equipment.

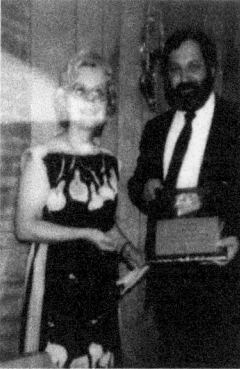

Lydia Havard

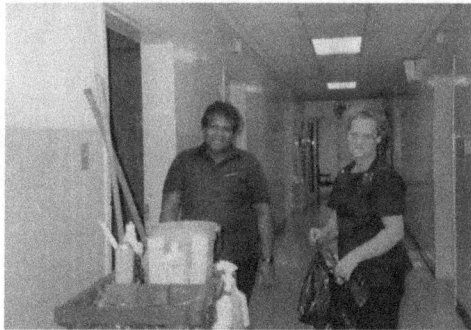

Leola Silas and Mary Fairley

Purchasing/Materials Management

By Deryk Parker

According to former employees with knowledge of the hospital, Corrine Morgan was one of the early materials managers for the hospital. Others who have been a part of that department have been Andy Haines and Mike Henderson along with Patsy Smith, who managed the department from 1990 to 1991.

Her son Alan Smith replaced her in that role and he was succeeded by Lendon Elmore as the overseer.

Deryk Parker was hired in November of 1994 to manage the department. He remained the manager until 2008.

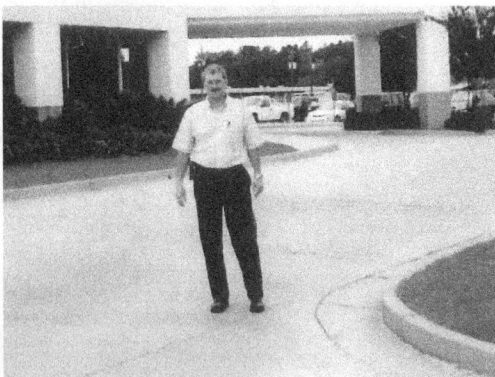

Deryk Parker

Auxiliary: "Pink Ladies" Caring for our Community for Decades

By Stephanie Chisholm

Although the exact formation date may not be easy to define, the important job of hospital volunteers has been felt by our patients and their families for years. Records indicate the Auxiliary of "Pink Ladies", as they are called because of the pink jackets they proudly wear, was originally formed in the mid to late 1970s.

A 1991 feature article in the George County Times names Stella Loftin and Lydia Havard as charter members, who were still active over 20 years later. In 1991, Johnnye Taylor, Auxiliary president, lead 14 active members. "We're here as a supportive element for the hospital. We help comfort patients and their families." And the mission has never changed.

Current records indicate the present-day Auxiliary began on August 6, 1998 with 23 volunteers. Twenty years later, six of the original members still serve: Faye McNeil, Doris Alexander, Rose Burgess, Mavis Dungan, Coe Alice Stirgus, and JoAnn Weaver.

In 1998, the Auxiliary was reestablished by Millie Wilhite and Linda Holland. In a newspaper interview in 1998, Ms. Wilhite explains, "George County Auxiliary is dedicated to provide the best volunteer services in supporting the activities of George County Hospital. Our goals are to promote the positive role of volunteers serving the hospital and to increase public awareness of the auxiliary membership and its role in the hospital to make it a sought-after activity in the community."

Shortly after its formation, Faye McNeil took the reins as president and still holds that title today. She's led the volunteers who selflessly give their time and energy five days a week. "It's a blessing being able to help the doctors and nurses with their patients." Faye adds. "And the hospital makes us feel so special. They feed us a wonderful meal each day, provide us with free flu shots, and we have a special luncheon every April."

The volunteers have many jobs throughout the hospital, from assisting patients and families to different departments throughout the hospital, to delivering flowers, to serving coffee as families wait for their loved ones, and even supplying pediatric patients with toys and coloring books. Auxiliary members average 550 volunteer hours each month.

Throughout its history, Auxiliary members have raised thousands of dollars for much-needed equipment and services which have touched thousands of patients and their families. Over the years, they've hosted community gospel sings, barbecue dinners, formal galas, bake sales, book fairs, and they've sold cookbooks to raise funds.

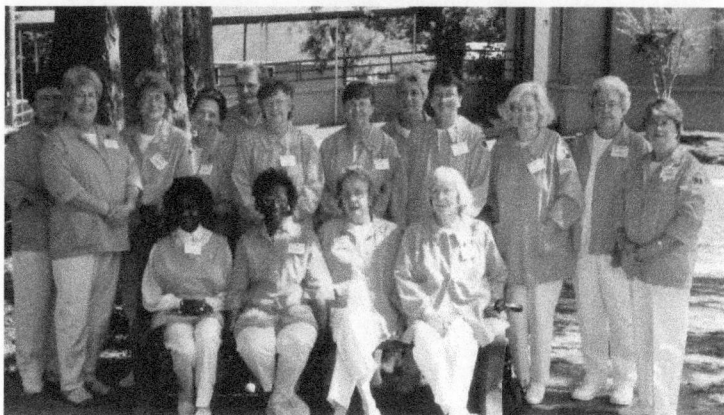

Seated L-R: CoAlice Sturgis, Doris Alexander, Nellie Dean Horn, Merle Tilley

Standing L-R: Joanne Weaver, Josie Henderson, Winnie Dale, Genora Brown, Rose Burgess, Mavis Dungan, Faye McNeill, Jean Persons, Laura Ballow, unknown, Lena Wozencraft, Margaret Graham

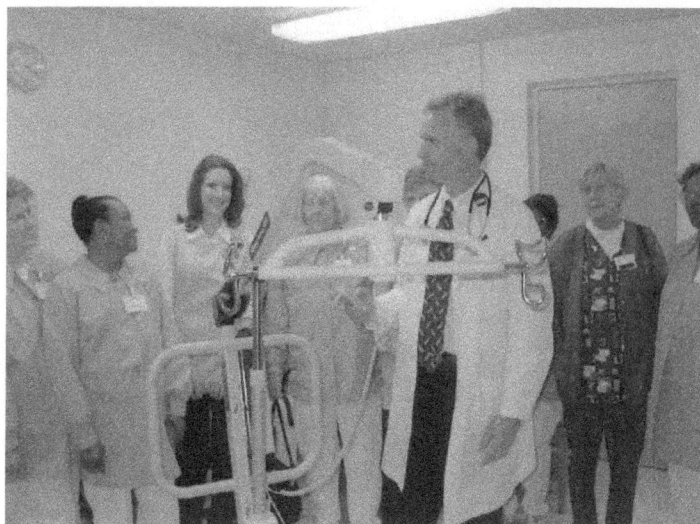

L-R: Melva Sidden, Carrie Jackson, Merle Tilley, Mark Scott, Jean Persons, Doris Alexander

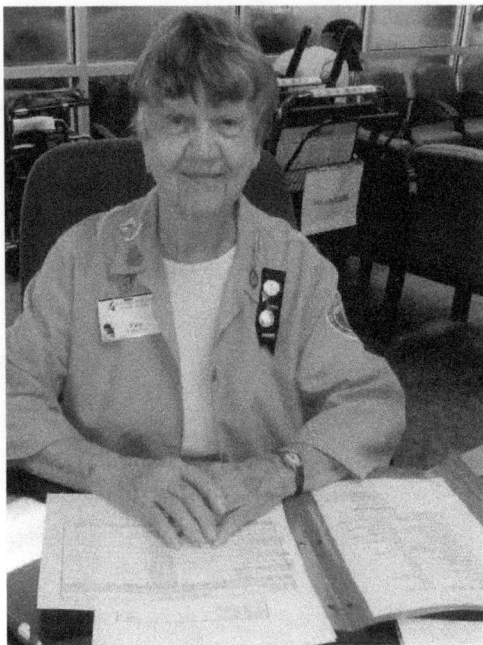

Faye McNeil

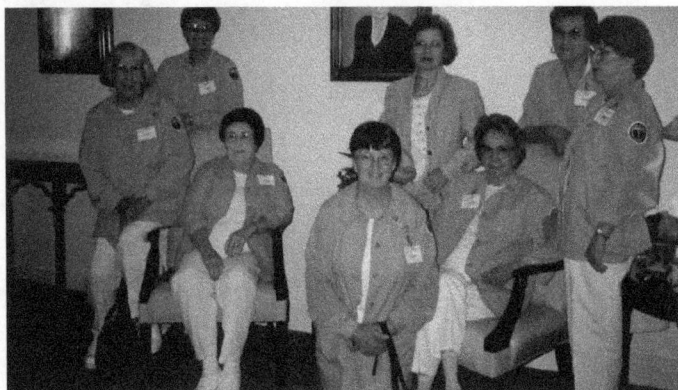

L-R: Merle Tilley, Laura Barrow, Joanne Weaver, Faye McNeil, Dimple Lollis, Nellie Dean Horn, Rose Burgess, Margaret Graham

...and a few more pictures!

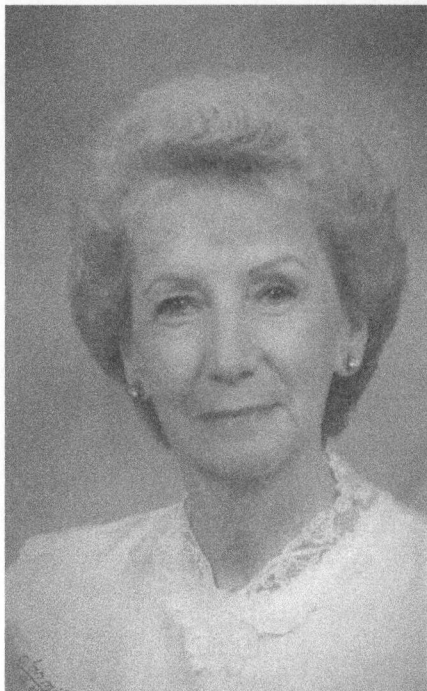

Regina Gunter

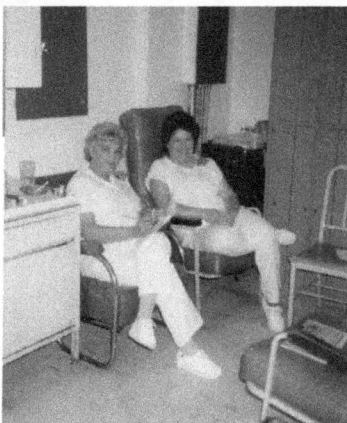

Shirley Thompson and Mary White

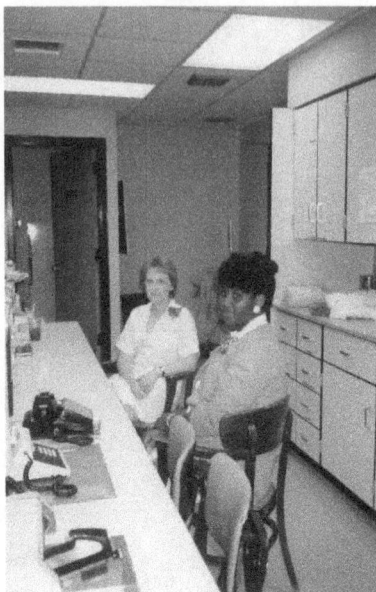

Millie Holt and Larita Hill

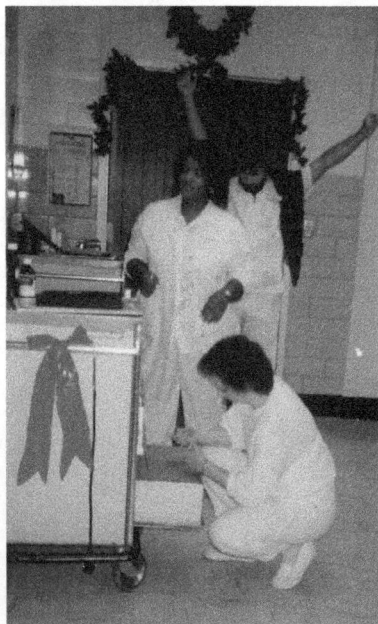

Back to front:
Paul May, Mae Bolton, Beth Mizell

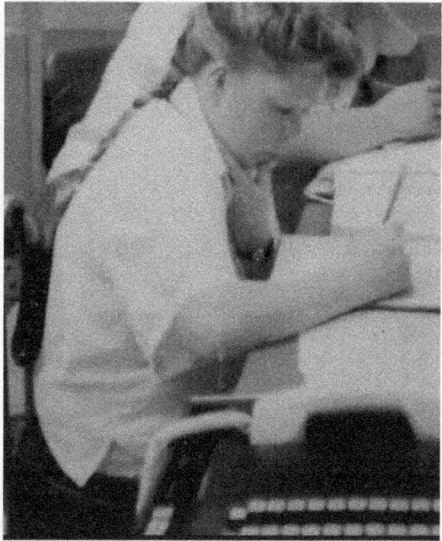

right: Kim Thomasson

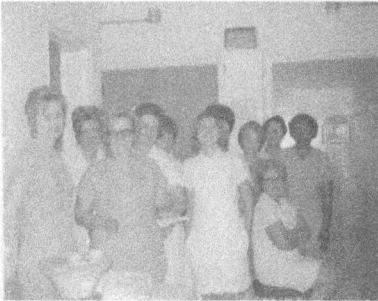

L-R: Sherry Gammage, Kathy Nell Griffin, Nell Cooley, Betty Bradley, Susan turner, Charlotte Davis, unknown, Jamie Boone, Rosemary Pankratz, Izola Miles, sitting: Doris Pope

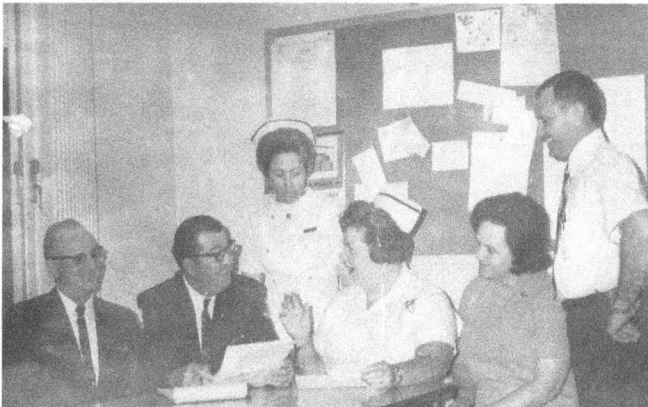

Rev. Bill Baggett, Al Rouse, Lena Wozencraft, Freida Davis, Willene Johnson, Johnny Mills

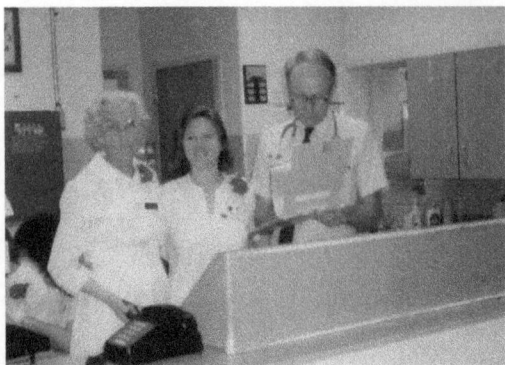

L-R: Annis Shaw, Shirley Miller, Dr. Whites

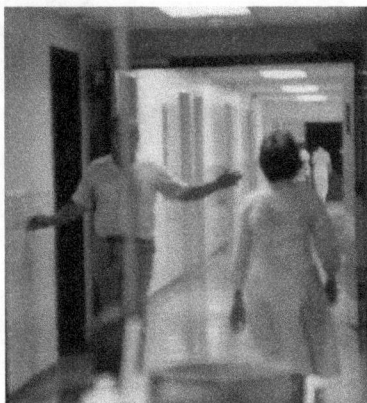

Benny Wall and Joyce Cochran

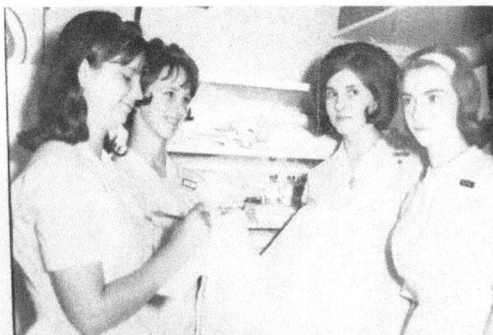

Early Candy Stripers, L-R: Glenda Chandler,
Pat Cook Havard, Brenda Marshall Underwood

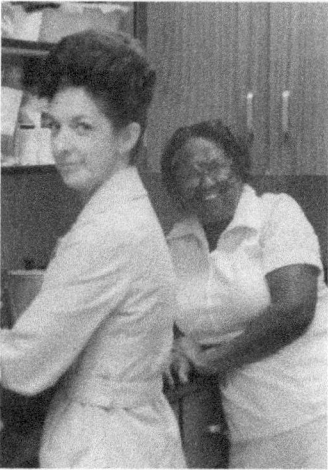

Eloise Bradley Farish and Lucille Lawrence

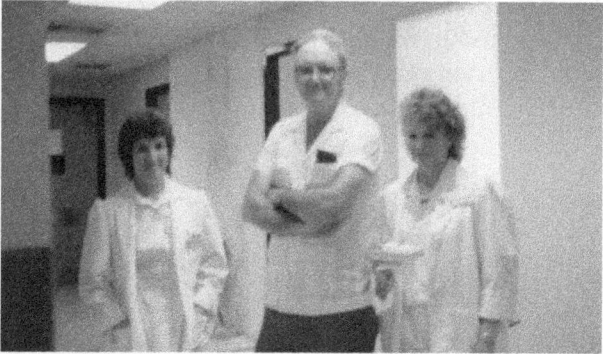

L-R: Eloise Bradley Farish, Gerald Evans, Joyce Rutherford

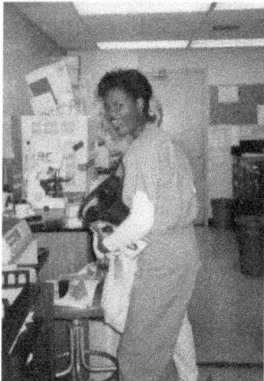

Angela Burkett

Epilogue

What began as a small community hospital fifty years ago has grown into a 48-bed hospital which continues to expand and modernize. And although the size of the facility has changed, one thing remains the same—that feeling of 'family' our patients experience while in our care.

We are proud of our rich history of supporting the community and are thrilled we've been successful in our mission of serving the healthcare needs of George County and the neighboring region.

I remember...

"I remember" by Christine Davis

I remember 2 episodes during my ambulance driving days:

Once when I was on driving duty, we had a patient that needed to be transferred to Mobile Infirmary. Dianne Miller was riding shot gun. (Actually riding in back taking care of the patient). The patient's condition warranted running with the lights flashing.

I noticed when we were in the vicinity of Crichton in Mobile, we were picked up by an escort with red lights flashing. The escort led us to the hospital. As we unloaded our patient, the nice fellow assisted and proceeded with us into the emergency entrance. Inside, the four of us were delayed waiting for a vacant bed. One of the Mobile Infirmary security officers accompanied us. When we had safely delivered our patient to his bed, Dianne and I thanked everyone for their help and returned to George County.

Later that evening, I received a call from the same Mobile Infirmary security officer inquiring if I had seen the local evening news. I told him I had not and he proceeded to tell me that the "officer" that escorted us earlier that day was later involved in a shoot-out with law enforcement on Dauphin Island Parkway. He was currently incarcerated at the Mobile Metro Jail.

He was charged with murdering a man in New Orleans and stealing his car. All I could say was "Oh my Lord!"

Not only had he posed as our police escort, I also discovered he had stolen my wallet from my purse in the ambulance. My wallet was also in New Orleans along with all the other "evidence". After several unsuccessful attempts to retrieve my wallet, I asked our local police if they would intercede for me with law enforcement in Mobile because I really needed my wallet. They agreed and eventually my wallet was returned.

On another occasion, we received a call that an 18-wheeler and an automobile had collided at the west end of the Chickasawhay River bridge. One of the drivers had been ejected into the river. As I was assessing the situation, trying to determine how to gain access to the patient in the car, a highway patrolman behind me said "you are going to have to crawl under that truck". I told him that I was sort of afraid to do that. He then said he would go with me. "Well, okay".

So, we proceeded to crawl under the truck and reach the injured man. We assessed, applied a cervical collar, got him on a backboard and proceeded to crawl back under the truck toward the ambulance, our patient in tow. Apparently, no one was directing traffic, because I noted as we emerged from under the truck, at least a dozen 18-wheelers end to end on this bridge. I remember thinking, "now how much weight will this bridge support?" This was another scary situation.

"I remember" by Joyce Rutherford

Joyce Cochran—walking briskly through the hall of the hospital, always smiling and singing joyfully as she carried cups of coffee to patients.

Mr. Benny Wall—always willing to stop from his busy day to share some of his wisdom with you over a cup of coffee

Lucille Lawrence—working silently and diligently in the Lab. It was back when we performed tests by hand---an order would come in for a particular test and by the time you got back from collecting the blood sample, Lucille had the reagents down from the shelf, the proper pipettes needed, etc. She would often bring you a fresh cup of coffee, fixed just like you liked it---even though you didn't ask for it. She really spoiled us. That's why we loved her so.

Dr. Dayton Whites and Dr. Tom Shaw---working day and night to take care of our medical community. It seemed that they had no other life. I'm not sure when they slept.

Annis Shaw, Helen Allen, Lena Rae Wozencraft, Regina Gunter---making sure that patients were given the best quality care possible.

Lavonia Hickman, Rosa Goff, and Madge Viguerie—wearing those crisp white dresses, complete with nurses' caps. They were also that meticulous about their work as LPNs.

Jake Rounsaville, Selma Patterson, Gladys Mercer, Marcella Leggett and others—working diligently as Aides, doing the dirty work to take care of patients--but maintaining a great attitude. It was a calling.

Lillie Maude Williams, Georgia Mae Ludgood, Mae Ruth Hill and others---working tirelessly in the kitchen to make those awesome meals for patients and staff. Lillie Maude was our staff meteorologist---she was terrified of bad weather!

J.C. and Gussie Jack---also working quietly and diligently—doing whatever was asked of them.

Christmas caroling on the front steps of the hospital.

Egg sandwiches for breakfast from the snack bar trailer in front of the hospital---so good!

Fried chicken day in the hospital cafeteria—we all looked forward to it!

"I remember" by Patsy Smith

When music was played in the hallways each day until visiting hours were over at 9pm. Dr Tipton came lots of nights and we would see who could name the most songs.

When you called the hospital and a person would answer the phone, "George County Hospital, may I help You?". Those were the days you actually talked to a person, not listened to an answering machine.

Parking between the two wings in back of the hospital beneath a large oak tree. Employees entered behind the first nurses' desk.

Coming to work because you loved your job and loved the hospital. We felt it was a privilege to be an employee of George County Hospital.

Employees singing Christmas carols on the front steps of the hospital. Dr. Tipton singing, "I'll have a blue Christmas".

Trying to pay the bills and make payroll. Going to check the mail to see how many payment checks were received for the day and what vendors could be paid.

Everyone knew everyone that worked at the hospital. When one hurt, we all hurt and when someone had a special something, we were all happy for them.

So many people I had the privilege of working with over the years. Registered Nurses: Maggie Parker, Jeanie Brewer, Lavelle McDerment, Annie V. Hillman, Nettie Reeves, Alice Hinton.

LPNs: Maude Whitsett, Lessie Long, Sybil Sumrall, Lille Bell Brotus Harrison, Juanita Stringfellow, Harlene Howell.

Nurse Aides: Katherine Whittington, Myrtle Moss, Mary Campbell, Etta Mae Reeves, Lula White.

Housekeeping: Joyce Pitts, Kathleen Todd, Leola Silas, Mary Fairley, Lucille Nix, Carrie Jackson, Gussie Jack, Daniel Sellers.

Orderlies: Dave Sylvester, Milton Armstrong, Jerry Hinton, Doye May, Clyde Blackston.

Dietary: Sharon Tipton, Obby Howell, J.J. Riley, Evelyn Prescott.

Business Office:

Lexie Solomon, Marie Weaver McEachern, Nancy Weaver Barrow, Lee Ann McMahon, Jan Harvey, Charlotte Brockway, Theresa Middleton, Debra Hancock, Ann Pipkins, Shana Moye, Sherry Williamson, Amy Goff, Missy Strahan, Boo White, Katie Goff, Deborah Dickson, Phyllis Howell, Betty Sue Weaver, Paul Scott, Kaye Rogers Howard, Willa Box, Karen Danley, Betty Knight, Angie Evans, Chestine O'Neal, Debbie Howell.

It seems the hospital always pulled through the hard times and survived to be the healthcare facility it is today. A hospital we can be thankful for that serves George County and the surrounding areas.

"I remember" by Dr. Dayton Whites

When the Hintons, registered nurse Hinton and orderly husband worked 11 to 7 shift and rode the Gulf Transport bus to work every night and rode back home to Hinton-ville each morning.

In 1961 to 1965 when the census was low, private patients were moved to semiprivate rooms at night and the second nurses station was closed. In the a.m. the private patients were moved back to their private rooms.

Ruby Bishop a night registered nurse who enjoyed waking physicians at night so much that she could not talk to the doctor for laughing at him because he was sleepy.

Joyce Cochran singing hymns to patients while giving respiratory treatments.

When you could ask pharmacy for aspirin, Tylenol or Benadryl and they would give it to you.

When you could get an x-ray or lab test without going through the outpatient department.

When all sixty beds in the hospital were occupied and patients were placed in the halls and waiting room.

When private rooms were $12.50 per day and semiprivate rooms were $10 per day. Also emergency room charges were $1.50 per visit.

When a trailer was placed behind the hospital and used as quarters for the emergency room physician. Physicians were paid $25 per hour.

When Ms. Sanderson rocked the newborn babies to sleep.

When all medical staff physicians made rounds twice a day. Sometimes morning rounds were started at 6am.

Sweet, sweet Mrs. Mary Ellen Rouse who was super nice to patients and always apologized to the local physician for bothering him for an order.

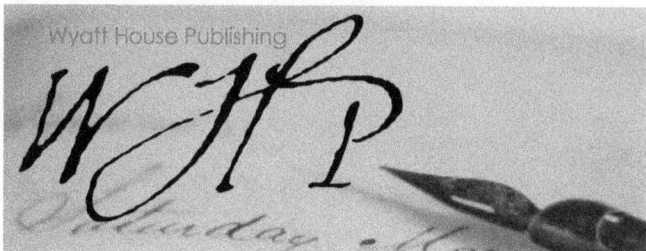
Wyatt House Publishing

You have a story.
We want to publish it.

Everyone has as a story to tell. It might be about something you know how to do, or what has happened in your life, or it may be a thrilling, or romantic, or intriguing, or heartwarming, or suspenseful story, starring a cast of characters that have been swimming around in your imagination.

And at Wyatt House Publishing, we can get your story onto the pages of a book just like the one you are holding in your hand. With professional interior design and a custom, professionally designed cover built just for you from the start, you can finally see your dream of being an author become reality. Then, you will see your book listed with retailers all over the world as people are able to buy your book from wherever they are and have it delivered to their home or their e-reader.

So what are you waiting for? This is your time.

visit us at

www.wyattpublishing.com

for details on how to get started becoming a published author right away.

www.ingramcontent.com/pod-product-compliance
Lightning Source LLC
Chambersburg PA
CBHW021934190326
41519CB00009B/1017